EYE EMERGENCIES

EYE EMERGENCIES

MICHAEL J. ROPER-HALL

ChM FRCS

Consultant Surgeon, Birmingham and Midland Eye Hospital;
Honorary Consultant Ophthalmic Surgeon,
The Queen Elizabeth Hospital and General Hospital, Birmingham;
Senior Clinical Lecturer and Tutor in Ophthalmology,
The Medical School, University of Birmingham, UK

Illustrations by Russell C. J. Kightley
Health Education Unit, Department of Ophthalmology,
Clinical Sciences Building, Leicester Royal Infirmary, UK

CHURCHILL LIVINGSTONE
EDINBURGH LONDON MELBOURNE AND NEW YORK 1987

CHURCHILL LIVINGSTONE
Medical Division of Longman Group UK Limited

Distributed in the United States of America by
Churchill Livingstone Inc., 1560 Broadway, New York,
N.Y. 10036, and by associated companies, branches
and representatives throughout the world.

First published 1987

ISBN 0-443-03269-6

British Library Cataloguing in Publication Data
Roper-Hall, M. J.
    Eye emergencies.
    1. Eye – Diseases and defects
    I. Title
    617.7'026   RE48

Library of Congress Cataloging in Publication Data
Roper-Hall, Michael J.
    Eye emergencies.

    Includes index.
    1. Ophthalmologic emergencies.   2. Eye – Wounds and
injuries.   I. Title.   [DNLM: 1. Emergencies.
2. Eye Diseases. 3. Eye Injuries.   WW 525 R784e]
RE48.R67   1987   617.7'026   86-24489

Produced by Longman Singapore Publishers (Pte) Ltd.
Printed in Singapore

PREFACE

Increasingly, eye emergencies and acute conditions present themselves to the accident and emergency departments of general hospitals. Some are simple and can be treated then and there. Others require referral for further management.

This book should help doctors, nurses and first-aid attendants without formal ophthalmic training, to examine, assess and understand the management of these ophthalmic conditions. Early in their training, ophthalmic House Officers will find themselves on duty to receive casualties and they too should find this book a useful guide and reminder.

The Birmingham and Midland Eye Hospital has always had a heavy emergency workload, so the conditions mentioned in the text are frequently seen there, but present more rarely in less specialised units.

I wish to acknowledge the advice and help of all my Consultant colleagues at the Birmingham and Midland Eye Hospital, in particular that of Miss Elizabeth Eagling, who read all the material during its preparation and assisted the development of its final form. Churchill Livingstone have been encouraging throughout and introduced me to Russell Kightley whose illustrations greatly enhance and lighten the text. It has been a pleasure to work with them all.

Birmingham, 1987   M. J. R.–H.

CONTENTS

Introduction

This book is intended for staff with little ophthalmic training, working in units which receive accidents and emergencies of all kinds. Among these there will be eye conditions in which the early management is all-important. They may present at First Aid points or in Accident and Emergency (A&E) departments and will include traumatic and non-traumatic acute conditions.

Some important facts have been intentionally repeated in different sections where appropriate to act as a reminder and to avoid the need for frequent cross-references.

Many minor conditions present to A&E departments and are mentioned so that they may be recognised, quickly differentiated from the important emergencies and managed without onward referral.

SERIOUS OR MINOR?

The most important task is to differentiate between serious and minor problems; those which require immediate attention and those which can safely wait. The casualty officer or general practitioner can be expected to see and treat minor conditions, and recognise serious conditions and refer them.

Patients requiring resuscitation, control of bleeding and stabilisation must have immediate attention to these vital problems. After this, perforating eye injuries should be allocated a high priority, higher than faciomaxillary fractures, simple limb fractures and suturing of most lacerations. Frequently, the ophthalmic injury is given low priority, but in the long term the patient's major disability is impaired vision.

ATTENDANCES

Trauma is the commonest single cause of attendance for ophthalmic conditions in the A&E department. Patients will also come because of impairment of vision, the acute onset of a red eye, ocular pain, or inflammation around the eye. Impairment of vision includes any diminution of acuity or field, blurring, floaters, flashes of light, double and sometimes multiple images.

CHEMICAL BURNS

Chemical burns claim the utmost priority, because a few moments can make the difference between saving sight and blindness. The emergency nature of a chemical burn must be known by everyone concerned. Some chemical agents can penetrate within seconds and continue to burn progressively.

HAZARDS

Hazards are constantly changing: as soon as one is removed, another predominates. A recent example is the effect of seatbelt legislation on trauma admissions to ophthalmic units. Before this legislation, eye injuries resulting from car accidents were common. Bilateral perforating injuries of the eyes with multiple facial lacerations resulted from passengers being thrown into a toughened glass windscreen. Wearing a seatbelt prevents this terrible injury. Assault and sports injuries are now more common reasons for admission.

Among children, a new craze can bring with it unexpected dangers, which may present in epidemic form. Whirlers, which were small propellers stamped out of thin metal and projected into the air up a spiral rod, rotated very rapidly and caused a series of transverse perforating injuries of cornea and sclera; these blinding injuries ceased as soon as these dangerous toys were withdrawn. Injuries from improvised bows and arrows tend to present with increased frequency when a new series of 'The Adventures of Robin Hood' is being shown.

Those working in A&E departments may be the first to realise the danger. They should be alert to the possibility of an increase of such injuries and be prepared to take steps towards their prevention.

PREVENTION OF DISABILITY

Once injury has occurred, prevention of disability depends upon the efficiency of ophthalmic management. Many injuries which could lead to blindness can now be treated more effectively. Particular progress has been made in safe and accurate closure of corneal wounds, surgery for traumatic cataract, vitreous haemorrhage and retinal detachment. Effective treatment of these conditions needs an experienced surgical team using special equipment. In serious cases, simple dressing at the place of injury should be followed by rapid transfer to a properly equipped treatment centre.

ACUTE BLINDNESS

Sudden loss of vision can be caused by vascular obstruction or haemorrhage in the eye or affecting the visual pathways, acute glaucoma, toxic retinopathy and optic neuritis. Retinal detachment usually causes slower deterioration. Virulent infections can imminently threaten corneal transparency (e.g. gonococcus, Pseudomonas).

UNIQUE ATTRIBUTES OF THE EYE

The structure of the eye is extraordinary in that living tissues are endowed with transparency and accurate optics so that clear images can be formed on the light-sensitive retina. Good vision depends on the clarity of the ocular media (cornea, aqueous humour, crystalline lens and vitreous body). They must maintain an accurate anatomical relationship with the retina.

Most ocular tissues have little or no regenerative properties. Defence mechanisms, which are an advantage in the healing of other tissues and organs, can have a seriously adverse effect on the eye. It may be necessary to suppress them.

The intraocular pressure is kept within physiological limits by a complex mechanism of aqueous circulation. This is easily disturbed, either temporarily or permanently, by trauma. Injuries to the uveal tissues (iris, ciliary body and choroid) can induce in them an inflammation (uveitis) which can excite a similar destructive inflammation in the uvea of the uninjured eye (sympathetic ophthalmitis). Thus an injury to one eye can result in total blindness.

The clinician has a heavy responsibility when faced with an acute ophthalmic problem, but the ocular structures are amenable to direct examination. A careful history and examination using proper illumination and magnification should provide the diagnosis and indicate the management. The remaining sections of this book are intended to help in this task.

Flow Diagram 1.1

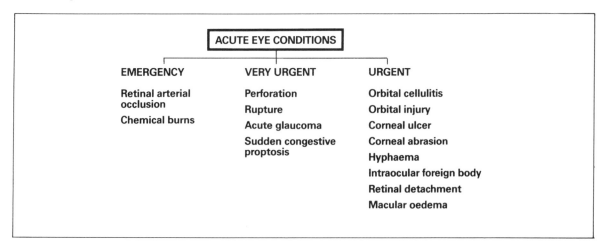

2

The effect of trauma on the eye

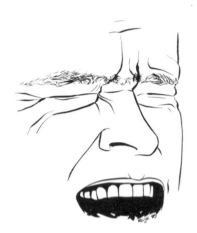

FORCES NEEDED TO CAUSE DAMAGE

The eye is highly specialised and vulnerable to a variety of injuries which are readily withstood by less complex tissues. The mechanical force needed to cause severe eye damage is of a different order from that in general trauma, and an injury sufficient to cause only a minor cut or bruise of an arm or leg may cause blindness of an eye.

In order to function the eye must be exposed, and this increases the possibility of accidental injury.

SAFEGUARDS

REFLEX RESPONSES

Some reactions to danger are instinctive. When trauma is threatened, the eyes are protected by dodging movements of the body and head, and the hands and arms are brought up to shield the impact. The blink reflex is rapid and is reinforced by tight closure of the eyelids, bringing a cushion of tissue about 1 cm thick in front of the eyes; at the same time the eyes rotate upwards, giving added protection (see Figure 2.1).

These protective reflexes are important in avoiding injury. They may, however, lose their relevance in conditions which present new hazards. For example, the eyes may be damaged by radiations which are invisible, causing no blink reflex, or so rapid that the reflex is too slow. A splash of molten metal or injurious chemical can enter the conjunctival sac, causing tight reflex closure of the lids, which after the event prolongs the effect of the agent and makes its removal much more difficult.

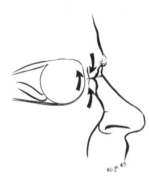

Fig. 2.1 Reflex protection of the eyes. Note how tight closure of the lids bunches up tissue in front of the globe. The eye rotates upwards, affording further protection to the cornea.

ANATOMICAL PROTECTION

Structurally the eye is protected by the lids and surrounded by a strong orbital margin, much of which is anterior to the globe. Within limits, the normal eye is capable of distortion without damage. It is supported on all sides and behind by a cushion of orbital fat (Fig. 2.2). The thin orbital wall nasally and below will give way if the force of injury is sufficient, reducing the trauma to the eye.

4

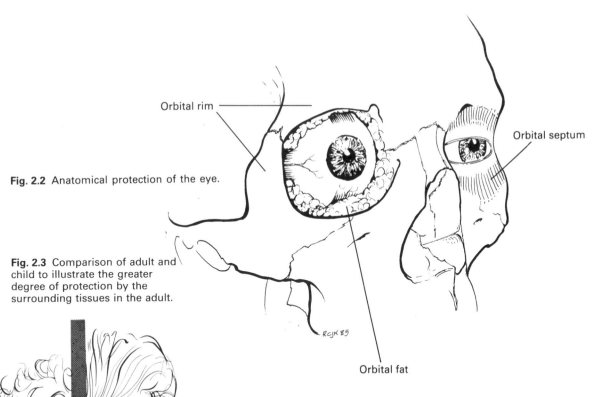

Fig. 2.2 Anatomical protection of the eye.

Fig. 2.3 Comparison of adult and child to illustrate the greater degree of protection by the surrounding tissues in the adult.

1½ years   25 years

CHILDREN AT RISK

Children are in special danger, because they are less aware of hazards and the child's eye is relatively less well protected because of the smaller orbit (Fig. 2.3). Paediatric eye injuries are often very severe, with a high incidence of perforating wounds. One-third of these lead to loss of the eye, so that there are more eyes lost during the first decade of life than at any other time. In the UK, this represents the loss by injury of one child's eye every day.

Children are especially vulnerable because they lack experience and can be led, unsuspecting, into danger by older children.

CLOSED LIDS CAN CAUSE LOSS OF VISION!

In a very young child with even a minor injury, short-term occlusion of the eye by lid swelling, or covering with a surgical dressing, can quickly cause blunting of vision (amblyopia).

ONE OR BOTH EYES?

Ocular injury is usually unilateral, but bilateral injury can occur in special circumstances.

It is not uncommon for one eye to be lazy (amblyopic) and, in the presence of unequal vision, injury to the good eye can be as disabling as a bilateral injury.

BILATERAL INJURY

By fire: when a patient is trapped or has lost consciousness
By a liquid chemical splash
By unseen radiations: in the ultraviolet and infrared range
By visible light: when outside physiological limits

Both eyes can be injured if the vulnerable person is unaware of danger because of:
1. Unconsciousness
2. Suddenness of the event

or if the patient is

3. Mentally handicapped
4. Uneducated
5. Uninstructed

and when

6. The danger is too sudden for natural protection, or
7. The forces are overwhelming.

PITFALLS FOR THE A&E DEPARTMENT

Here are examples of circumstances in which there is danger of delayed recognition of severe ocular damage. This may happen:
1. When it is difficult or unsafe to expose the eye
2. In the presence of other major injury which is given priority, and because
3. Deep injury is often less painful than superficial injury
4. The optic nerve is vulnerable with little overt evidence of damage
5. Signs may be minimal at first, but rapidly increase in severity.

WHEN IT IS DIFFICULT OR UNSAFE TO EXPOSE THE EYE

An eye injury is concealed soon after facial trauma by gross oedema or haematoma. Attempts at forcible opening may compound the damage to the eye. Judgement may have to be based on the history, deferring full examination until it can be carried out under general anaesthesia.

With a 'black eye' looking as if it affects the lids alone, there may be some permanent ocular lesion, which careful examination will reveal. An orbital fracture may be found with a more severe injury, but the concurrent contusion injury to the eye will not be obvious without slit-lamp or ophthalmoscopic examination. At first such examination would be impossible because of lid swelling.

IN THE PRESENCE OF OTHER MAJOR INJURY WHICH IS GIVEN PRIORITY

In multiple injury, lifesaving measures have to take priority, but the eyes must be protected and their integrity checked as soon as conditions permit.

DEEP INJURY IS OFTEN LESS PAINFUL THAN SUPERFICIAL INJURY

The corneal surface is extremely sensitive to pain, but deeper injury may be pain-free although more serious. It is all too easy for a perforating injury of the eye to be missed until secondary complications draw attention to it.

THE OPTIC NERVE IS VULNERABLE WITH LITTLE OVERT EVIDENCE OF DAMAGE

Concussion injury typically seen after a fall from a bicycle may be associated with shearing damage to the optic nerve and complete blindness of one eye. This is caused by tearing of the small vessels running into the optic nerve within the optic foramen (Fig. 2.4).

Fig. 2.4 Scheme showing blood supply to the optic nerve (right side, viewed laterally).

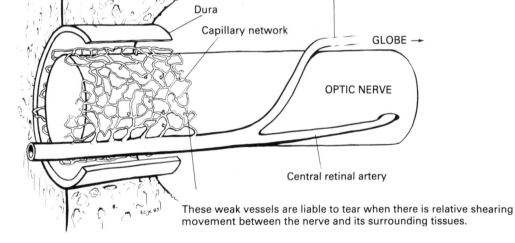

Bone around optic foramen

Dura

Capillary network

Ophthalmic artery

GLOBE →

OPTIC NERVE

Central retinal artery

These weak vessels are liable to tear when there is relative shearing movement between the nerve and its surrounding tissues.

There is no obvious abnormality in the fundus appearance until the nerve head shows atrophy some weeks later. An absent direct pupil reaction to light with a normal consensual reaction is the important early positive finding (afferent pupil defect).

SIGNS MAY BE MINIMAL AT FIRST, BUT RAPIDLY INCREASE IN SEVERITY

Virulent organisms may be present in the conjunctival sac and yet show no clinical sign. The presence of an intact corneal epithelium is all-important in preventing rapid and serious deeper infection. *Pseudomonas* infection of a burn represents a serious threat to the cornea of both eyes if the epithelium is damaged by exposure in a seriously ill or unconscious patient. The epithelium urgently needs protection from the drying effects of exposure.

Apparently localised infected lesions on the face and around the orbit can spread rapidly by thrombophlebitis into the deeper orbital tissues and the cavernous sinus (Fig. 2.5). Some chemical burns can abolish pain sensation, and a badly damaged cornea may still be surprisingly transparent soon after injury, becoming totally opaque within a few hours.

Fig. 2.5 Scheme of cavernous sinus.

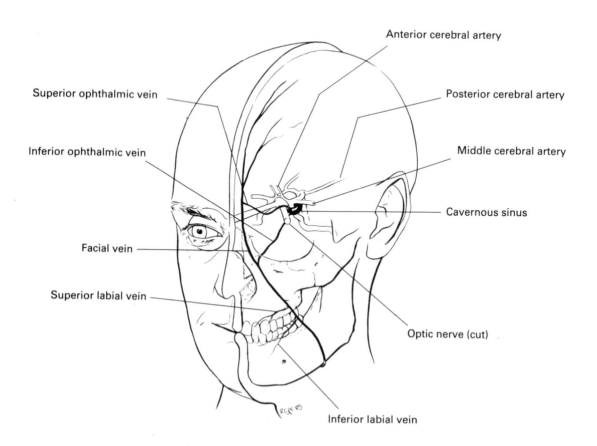

Symptoms and circumstances causing attendance at A & E departments

Flow Diagram 3.1

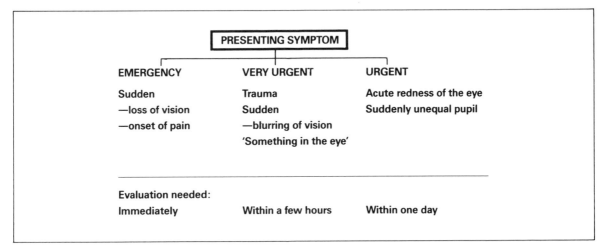

Most attendances will be in relation to:

1. Trauma affecting the eye and orbit
2. A red eye
3. Painful eye conditions
4. Loss of vision with or without pain

These will be briefly outlined, with reference to particular conditions. Presenting symptoms are analysed in Flow Diagram 3.1.

TRAUMA AFFECTING THE EYE AND ORBIT

Eye injuries are classified in Table 3.1. It should be noted that the adjacent structures need similar consideration.

Table 3.1 Classification of eye injuries

Mechanical	Non-mechanical
Superficial	Burns
Blunt	Thermal
Penetrating	Chemical
With intraocular foreign body	Radiational
Without intraocular foreign body	

The trauma may present as mainly an eye condition or combined with orbital or more remote multiple injury. If vision is affected in a conscious person, it is likely that he or she will give the eyes priority when seeking help. In an unconscious person with multiple and obvious injury, the presence of ocular damage is often overlooked. This may be because the eyes are concealed behind tightly closed lids.

It is not easy to obtain a clear and concise history in emergency situations, and inaccuracies may confuse management decisions later. When the emergency has passed, the history should be gone over again, perhaps with additional information from witnesses or relatives to correct errors.

Children should seldom be expected to give an accurate history.

SUPERFICIAL INJURIES

These are usually painful and associated with lacrimation and photophobia. They are described in more detail on page 71 et seq.

BLUNT INJURY

This can affect all ocular and surrounding structures. Damage to the external eye is usually obvious, but associated lesions may be concealed. See pages 70, 88, 93, 98.

PENETRATING INJURIES

These may not be obvious. In the eye, small penetrations may cause sufficient intraocular damage to threaten sight. The history is important, and a penetration should be suspected if a sharp object was involved. An intraocular foreign body is likely if the injury happened when a hand hammer was being used. See pages 91, 99.

BURNS

These may not be painful if they are deep enough to destroy pain nerve endings.

Thermal burns
These usually affect the eyelids and not the eye itself, unless the patient was unconscious or the accident happened without visible warning. The blink reflex is quick enough in most circumstances to protect the eye. See pages 76, 87, 102.

Chemical burns
These can cause permanent damage in seconds. Many alkalis can penetrate through and between the cells of the cornea to enter the anterior chamber and intraocular tissues before being neutralised. Acids may not cause such deep damage, because coagulation of the tissues prevents further penetration. See pages 88, 103.

Radiational burns

The common acute radiational burns are due to ultraviolet light. These happen after 'welding flash' and inadequate protection when using 'sunray lamps'. There is a latent period of a few hours without symptoms, then sudden and severe pain, lacrimation and photophobia. Because of the delayed symptoms, the patient may not give the history of exposure until asked directly.

A RED EYE

This is usually due to:
1. Visible haemorrhage
2. Inflammatory congestion
3. Vascular dilatation or venous embarrassment

Flow Diagram 3.2

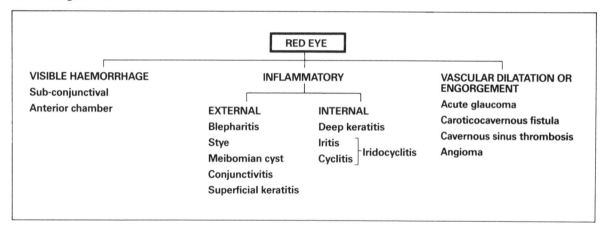

VISIBLE HAEMORRHAGE

Haemorrhage is visible when there is a sub-conjunctival haemorrhage or when there is bleeding into the anterior chamber.

Sub-conjunctival haemorrhages

These haemorrhages are obvious; the larger ones are prominent and will take longer to clear (Fig. 3.1).

It is necessary to differentiate between those of local origin and those resulting from fracture of the anterior cranial fossa or orbit. They can occur spontaneously or from injury, and the blood can conceal scleral damage, making it easy to miss an underlying perforation or rupture.

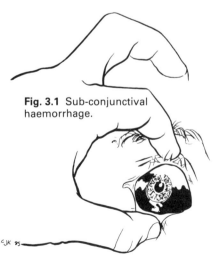

Fig. 3.1 Sub-conjunctival haemorrhage.

Blood in the anterior chamber (hyphaema)

Blood in the chamber may fill it; at first red, it becomes black with age or when the pressure in the eye is raised. If blood is not filling the chamber, a fluid level is soon evident in a resting patient, but commonly on arrival in the A&E department the blood is diffused throughout the chamber, making examination of the iris and lens impossible at that stage (see Figure 3.2).

Fig. 3.2 Blood in the anterior chamber (hyphaema).

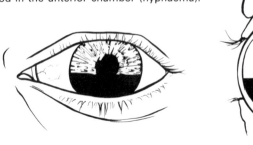

INFLAMMATORY CONGESTION

Inflammatory conditions of the eye are associated with vascular congestion with a distribution which indicates the affected structures.

Blepharitis

This shows mainly as redness of the lid margins, with crusting or more frank discharge (Fig. 3.3).

Fig. 3.3 Blepharitis.

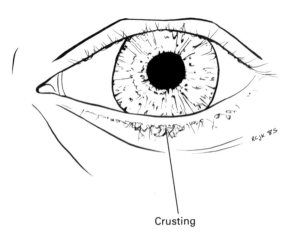

Crusting

Fig. 3.4 Stye (hordeolum).

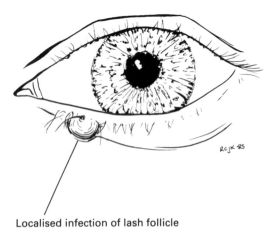

Localised infection of lash follicle

A stye (hordeolum)
This is a localised infection of a lash follicle or associated glands with local pain and tenderness (Fig. 3.4)

Meibomian cysts

These can have an acute onset with pain (meibomitis, hordeolum internum). The tenderness and swelling is in the tarsal plate away from the lid margin (Fig. 3.5). Sometimes many meibomian glands are infected, with inspissated secretion protruding from the duct orifices on the lid margin.

Fig. 3.5 Meibomian cyst.

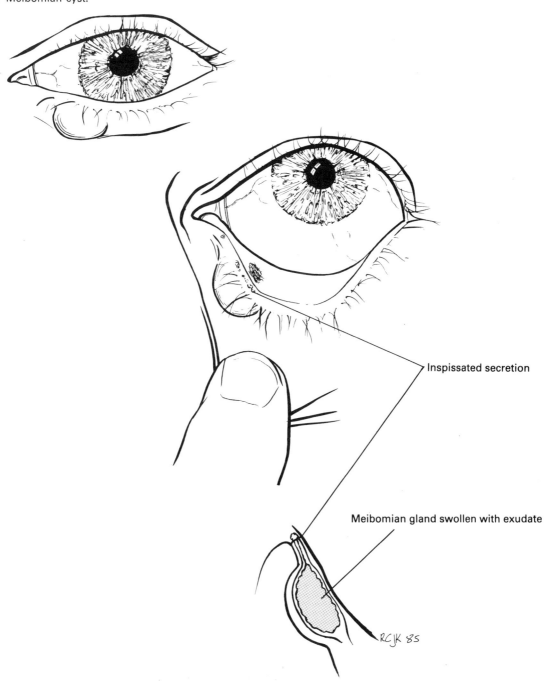

Inspissated secretion

Meibomian gland swollen with exudate

RCJK '85

Conjunctivitis

This usually exhibits congestion of the whole mucous membrane, but in certain forms it is more evident on the inner aspects of the lids, or at the angles (Fig. 3.6).

Fig. 3.6 Conjunctivitis.

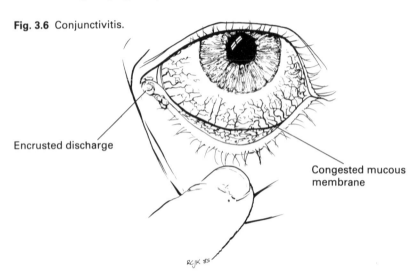

Encrusted discharge

Congested mucous membrane

Keratitis, iritis, cyclitis

Inflammation of the cornea (keratitis), iris (iritis) or ciliary body (cyclitis) is shown by a ring of congestion of the smaller and deeper vessels at the corneal margin (ciliary injection, or circumcorneal injection) (Fig. 3.7). Often both the iris and ciliary body are involved in the same inflammatory lesion (iridocyclitis).

Fig. 3.7 Circumcorneal injection.

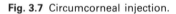
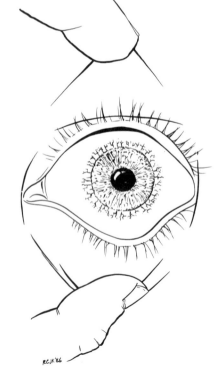

Congested vessels associated with inflammation of the nearby cornea/iris/ciliary body

Flow Diagram 3.3

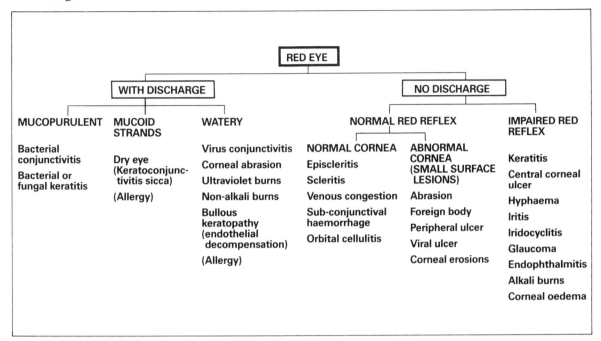

VASCULAR CONGESTION OR ENGORGEMENT

This is seen in acute glaucoma, also in caroticocavernous fistula, in cavernous sinus thrombosis in association with the angioma of the Sturge-Weber syndrome and as part of a generalised flush or congestion of the face.

Acute red eye conditions are differentiated in Table 3.2. See also Flow Diagrams 3.2 and 3.3.

Table 3.2 Red eye differential (excluding trauma)

	Conjunctivitis	Keratitis	Acute iritis	Acute Glaucoma
Onset	1–7 days	1–4 days	1–3 days	Today
Symptoms				
Vision	Normal	Reduced	Reduced	Severe loss
Pain	Gritty	Sharp	Moderate	Severe
Photophobia	No	Yes	Marked	Slight
Systemic	None	Little	Malaise	Vomiting prostration
Tenderness	No	Slight	Marked	Marked
Congestion	Red	Red at limbus	Red at limbus	Purple at limbus
Signs				
Discharge	Purulent	Watery	Watery	Watery
Pupil	Normal	Normal or smal!	Small, inactive	Fixed, dilated
Cornea	Normal	Opaque	Bright reflex	Steamy
Anterior chamber	Normal	Normal	Exudate	Shallow
Iris	Normal	Normal	Muddy, injected	Grey
Ocular pressure	Normal	Normal	Variable	Very high
Treatment				
	Antibiotic	See text, page 79	Mydriatic, steroid	Miosis, acetazolamide

PAINFUL EYE CONDITIONS

Patients may present with:

1. Lid tenderness with inflammatory conditions of the lids: stye, blepharitis, infected meibomian cyst.

2. Pain on movement of the eye: retrobulbar neuritis, subtarsal foreign body, corneal foreign body, corneal abrasion, recurrent corneal abrasion, scleritis, periocular inflammation.

3. Pain referred to the eye: sinusitis, herpes zoster ophthalmicus.

4. Pain in the eye: keratitis, corneal abrasion, ulcer or foreign body, acute iritis, acute glaucoma.

The combination of pain, loss of vision and a red eye is serious and should indicate referral to an ophthalmologist. Even without loss of vision, a painful red eye may also threaten sight.

LOSS OF VISION WITH OR WITHOUT PAIN

The conditions which present with visual impairment are tabulated in the following flow diagrams. The first (Flow Diagram 3.4) considers the differential diagnosis related to the presence or absence of pain.

Flow Diagram 3.4

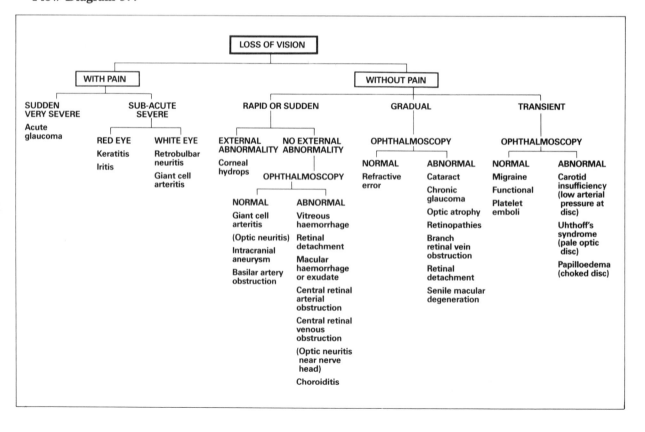

Pupil reactions can be helpful in the assessment of patients without other obvious signs.

Flow Diagram 3.5

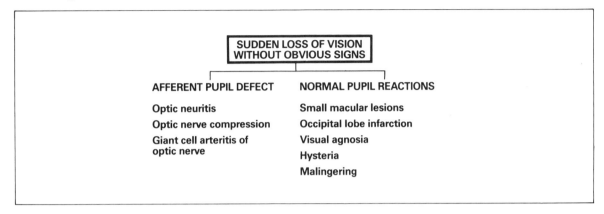

Blurred vision is a common presenting symptom, which may affect one or both eyes. It is helpful to differentiate between causes of sudden and gradual onset, and by observing the quality of the red reflex.

Flow Diagram 3.6

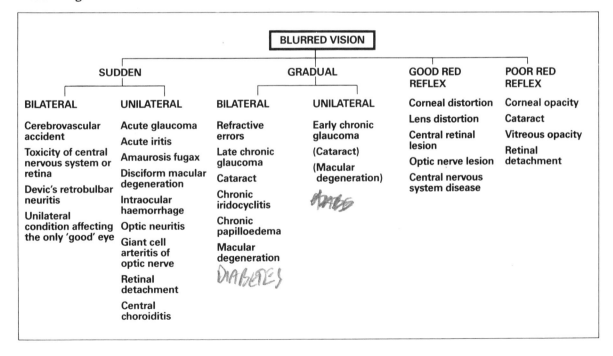

4

History, examination and preliminary assessment

Following injury, different conditions apply from other acute presentations. History taking and the sequence of examination differ sufficiently for them to be considered separately. Non-traumatic cases are discussed on page 55.

AFTER TRAUMA

HISTORY

Take a concise but accurate history, recording:
– time of injury
– circumstances of accident
– nature of causative agent
– immediate action taken
– subsequent first aid
– previous ophthalmic history
  Check whether spectacles or contact lenses are normally worn.
  Remember that patients often forget a previous history of eye problems, such as a squint or lazy (amblyopic) eye, even when they are asked.
  Beware of accepting a history given by an injured child – it is often unreliable because of inaccurate description or fear of punishment.

EXAMINATION

1. Make the patient as comfortable as possible lying down or sitting with head support.
2. Have the following instruments to hand (see also page 68):
– an inspection torch
– an ophthalmoscope
– sterile gauze and cotton buds to assist lid opening.
3. Observe without touching:
– Does lid swelling prevent voluntary opening?
– Is there visible laceration or puncture wound?
– Is there blood or other debris between the lid margins?
Most patients can co-operate, but many instinctively and erroneously believe it will help the examination if the other eye is kept closed and the head turned away.

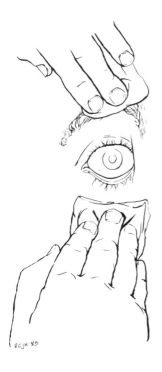

Fig. 4.1 Opening the eye without putting pressure on the globe.

4. Instruct the patient:
– to avoid protective squeezing which may lead to further damage to the eye
– to keep the head still.

Ask the patient when you are examining:
– to try to keep both eyes open
– to keep the hands away.

5. Explain to the patient what you are doing and that you will be as gentle as possible.

6. If the patient cannot open the eyes, assist by retracting the lids with gauze on the brow and cheek, avoiding pressure on the globe, because:
– the eye may be very tender
– pressure may cause prolapse or fresh bleeding.

See Figure 4.1.

7. Measure the visual acuity. Begin with the worst affected eye, covering the other.
– Is there light perception?
– Can the patient tell the direction from which the light is being shone? This can usually be done even through closed lids.
– If the lids are open, can he/she see hand movements?
– Can he/she count fingers, and from how far? (Estimate the distance up to 1 metre.)
– If fingers can be counted, proceed to use a Snellen's distance chart.
– If vision is sub-normal, test again with spectacles if these are available.
– If not, best vision can be estimated quite well by asking the patient to read the letters through a pin-hole aperture (Fig. 4.2).

Record the result.

Repeat the procedure with the other eye.

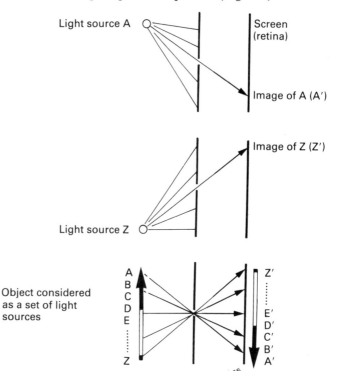

Fig. 4.2 Pin-hole effect.

Examination with the inspection torch

8. Inspect the lids more closely for bruising or laceration. Look for lid margin involvement.

9. Examine the eyes for injury. Help the patient to keep both eyes open. (Terminate further direct examination if there is any fresh bleeding. X-rays and other indirect tests may be necessary before the patient is taken to the operating theatre for further specialist examination and repair.)

a. Examine the cornea for laceration or opacity.
– How extensive is the lesion?
– Is the corneal margin or sclera involved? (See Figure 4.3.)

Fig. 4.3 Average corneal dimensions.

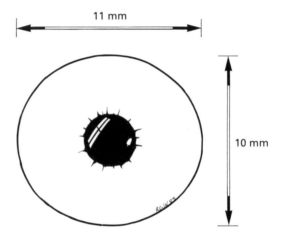

b. Compare the anterior chamber in both eyes.
– Is it shallow, or absent, in the injured eye?
– Does it contain blood? This is common in blunt injury indicating damage to vessels at the iris root. It soon sediments to form a fluid level (hyphaema). (See Figure 4.4.)

Fig. 4.4 Blood in the anterior chamber (hyphaema).

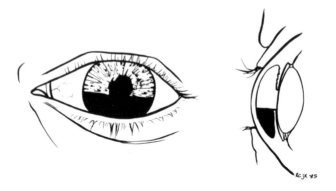

c. Inspect the iris.
- Is the pupil central?
- Is the pupil circular?
- Is the iris damaged behind a laceration? This may show as a tear, or displacement of the pupil. Prolapsed iris tissue usually loses its pigment and looks like a strand of exudate. See Figures 4.5, 4.6 and 4.7.

Fig. 4.5 Iris sphincter damage.

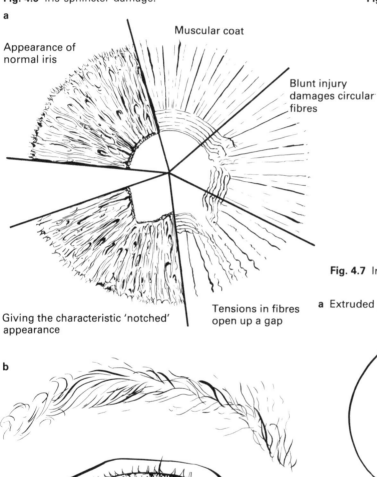

a

Appearance of normal iris

Muscular coat

Blunt injury damages circular fibres

Tensions in fibres open up a gap

Giving the characteristic 'notched' appearance

b

Observe 'notch' in red reflex

RCJK 85

Fig. 4.6 Dialysis.

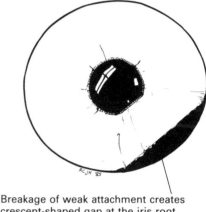

RCJK 85

Breakage of weak attachment creates crescent-shaped gap at the iris root. This is best seen with trans-illumination.

Fig. 4.7 Iris prolapse.

a Extruded portion of iris; tends to lose pigmentation

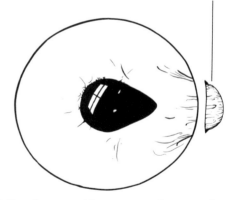

b Ballooning caused by pressure of aqueous humour

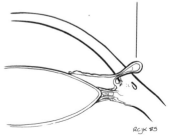

RCJK 85

If the pupil is undamaged, observe its reaction to direct light. Then observe its response when the other eye is stimulated (consensual). See Figures 4.8 and 4.9.

Fig. 4.8 Normal equal response.

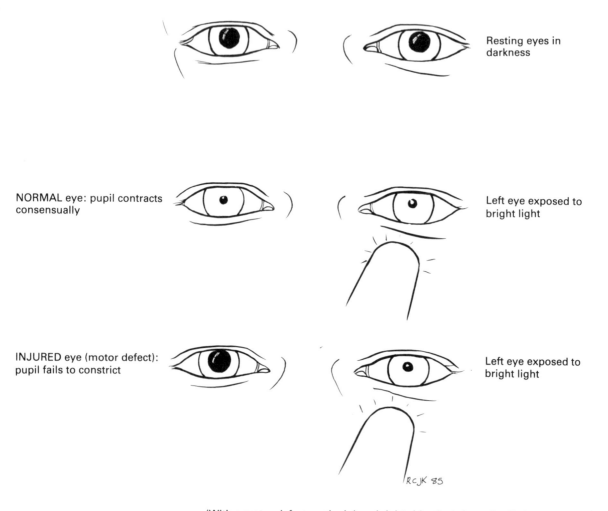

Resting eyes in darkness

NORMAL eye: pupil contracts consensually

Left eye exposed to bright light

INJURED eye (motor defect): pupil fails to constrict

Left eye exposed to bright light

RCJK 85

(With a motor defect on the injured right side, the left pupil will show a normal consensual reaction when the right eye is stimulated.)

d. Look within the pupil.
– Is the lens damaged? Lens cortex quickly becomes swollen and opaque if the capsule is torn (Fig. 4.10).
– Is it displaced? This can show as uneven depth of the AC, or tremulous lens or iris. See Figure 4.11.

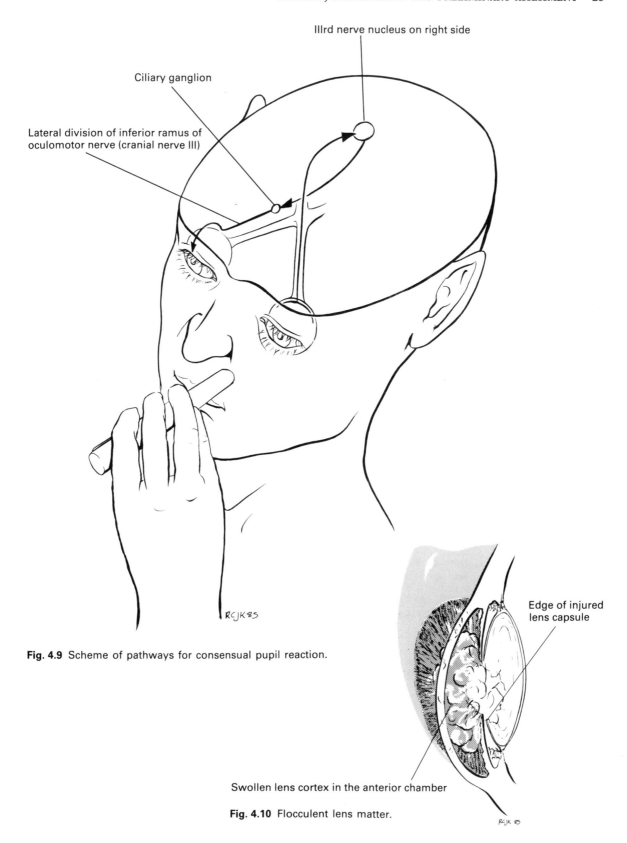

IIIrd nerve nucleus on right side

Ciliary ganglion

Lateral division of inferior ramus of
oculomotor nerve (cranial nerve III)

Fig. 4.9 Scheme of pathways for consensual pupil reaction.

Edge of injured
lens capsule

Swollen lens cortex in the anterior chamber

Fig. 4.10 Flocculent lens matter.

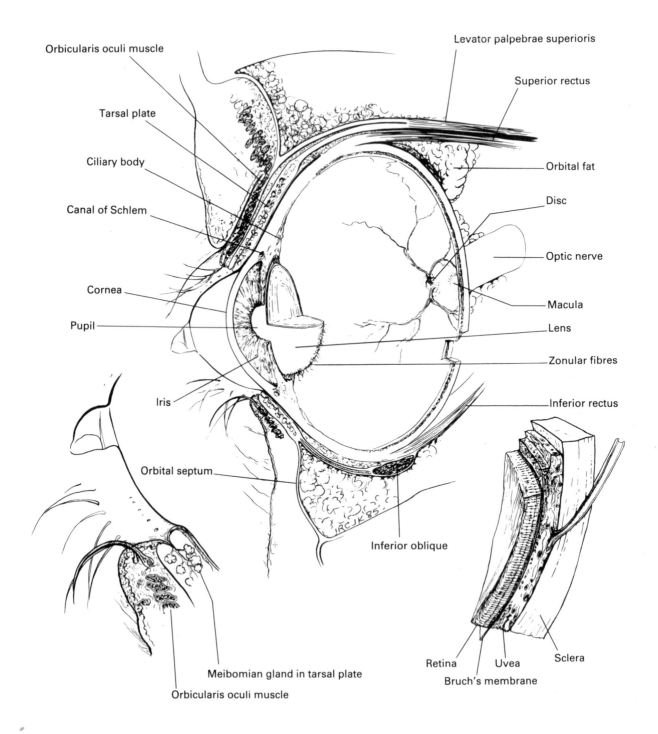

Fig. 4.11 Ocular anatomy (vertical section).

e. Examine the conjunctiva and sclera in each quadrant.
– Is there conjunctival laceration or haemorrhage?
– Does a haemorrhage have a defined posterior edge?
– Does this conceal a scleral laceration or rupture? Darker areas may indicate uveal exposure or prolapse. (See Figure 4.12.)
– Are the blood vessels engorged?

Record these findings.

Fig. 4.12 Sub-conjunctival bleeding masking a scleral wound.

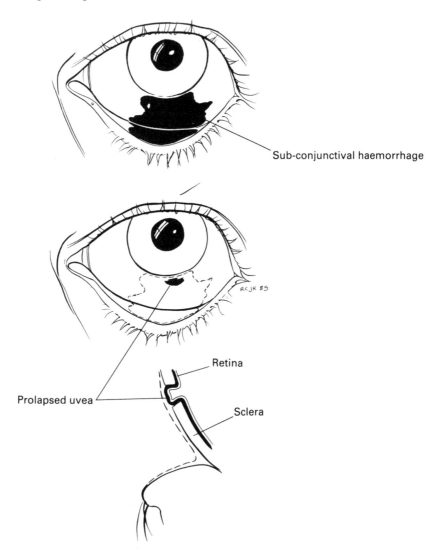

Sub-conjunctival haemorrhage

Retina

Prolapsed uvea

Sclera

Examination using the ophthalmoscope
Observe the pupil from 20–30 cm.
– Is the red reflex normal?
– If not, where is the opacity?

With the ophthalmoscope held 20–30 cm from the patient's face, the eye can be observed coaxial to the light beam and a red reflex is seen through the normal pupil. A grey or black opacity in the reflex is due to corneal or lens damage, blood or exudate in front of or *behind* the lens. A total opacity is probably due to vitreous haemorrhage. (See Figure 4.13.)

Fig. 4.13 Using parallax to locate intraocular features.

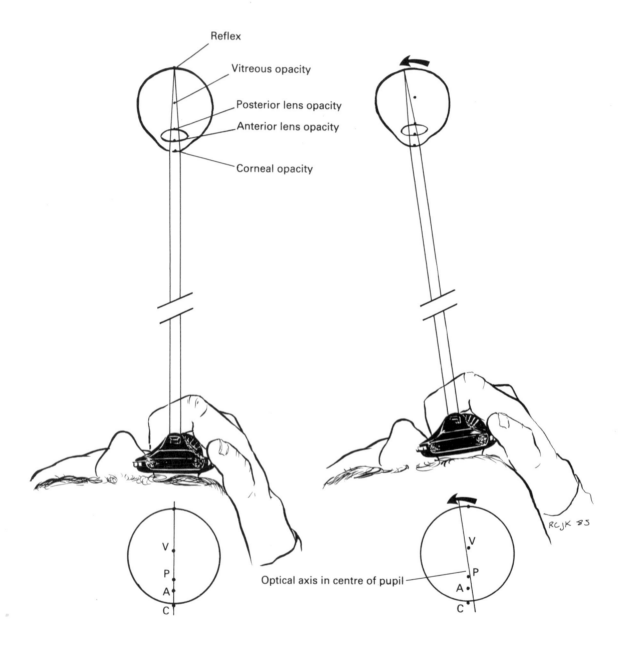

Reflex

Vitreous opacity

Posterior lens opacity

Anterior lens opacity

Corneal opacity

V
P
A
C

Optical axis in centre of pupil

V
P
A
C

Observer sees opacities behind pupil shift to the right, and in front of pupil to the left.

Now approach the eye more closely. Still observe through the pupil and focus the ophthalmoscope. If the red reflex is good, the fundus of the eye will be seen. Observe the:
- optic disc
- blood vessels
- general background
- macula

Retinal oedema appears as a white area, and blood, of course, is red, but often quite dark. A retinal break usually shows as red (the vascular choroid seen through the hole) surrounded by grey (the retina detached around it).

Record the findings.

Further examination

At this point examination of the visual fields may be needed. The method is described on page 57. In some cases a more complete neurological examination will be necessary. The ophthalmic examination can be completed by an evaluation of the co-ordination of ocular movements, examination of the ocular adnexae and a fuller assessment of lid and orbital damage.

The observation of head posture is easier with the patient sitting up.

Extraocular muscles (Fig. 4.14, 4.15, 4.16)

Fig. 4.14 The extraocular muslces.

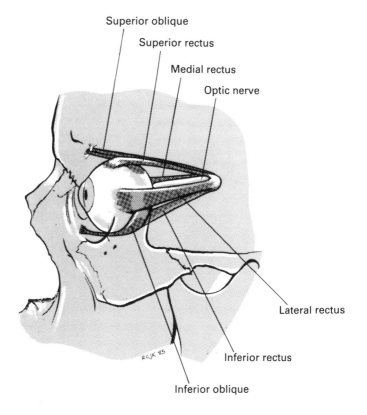

Superior oblique

Superior rectus

Medial rectus

Optic nerve

Lateral rectus

Inferior rectus

Inferior oblique

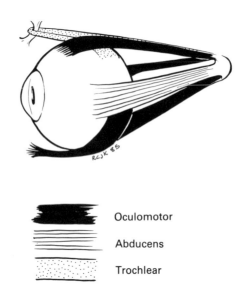

Oculomotor

Abducens

Trochlear

Fig. 4.15 Innervation of the extraocular muscles (left eye).

Fig. 4.16 Scheme of innervation of the extraocular muscles.

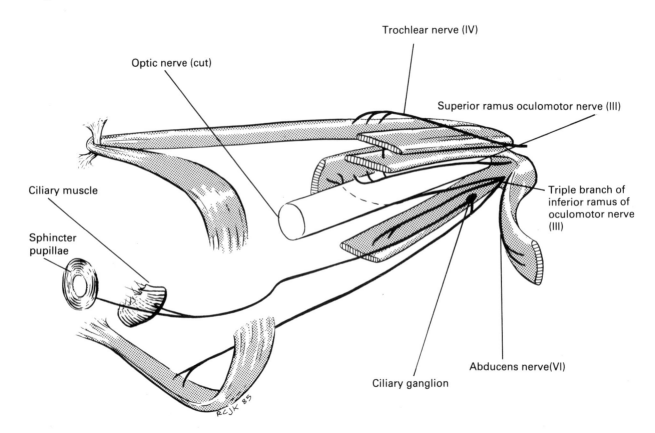

Observe the patient's posture.
– Does the patient have an abnormal head posture?

a. Third nerve palsy

Here the patient does not exhibit an abnormal head posture, because the affected side is occluded by ptosis of the upper lid (Fig. 4.17).

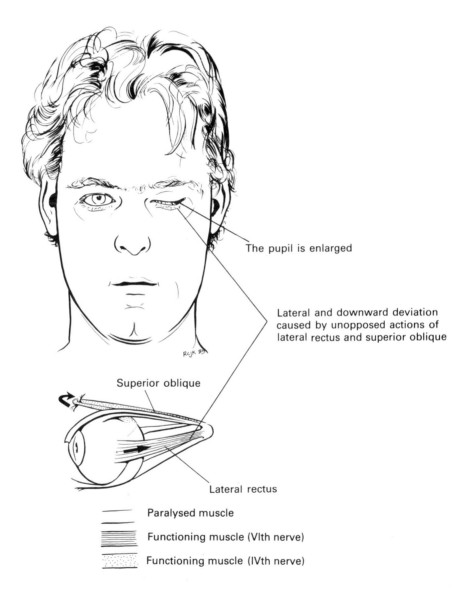

The pupil is enlarged

Lateral and downward deviation caused by unopposed actions of lateral rectus and superior oblique

Superior oblique

Lateral rectus

—— Paralysed muscle

≡≡≡ Functioning muscle (VIth nerve)

··· Functioning muscle (IVth nerve)

Fig. 4.17 IIIrd nerve palsy with ptosis and lateral deviation.

b. Fourth nerve palsy

Unilateral (Fig. 4.18):
This produces a gross tilt and turn of the head away from the affected side. The chin is dipped.

Bilateral (Fig. 4.19):
This shows the chin dipped to the chest.

Fig. 4.18 Unilateral IVth nerve palsy (left eye).

Fig. 4.19 Bilateral IVth nerve palsy.

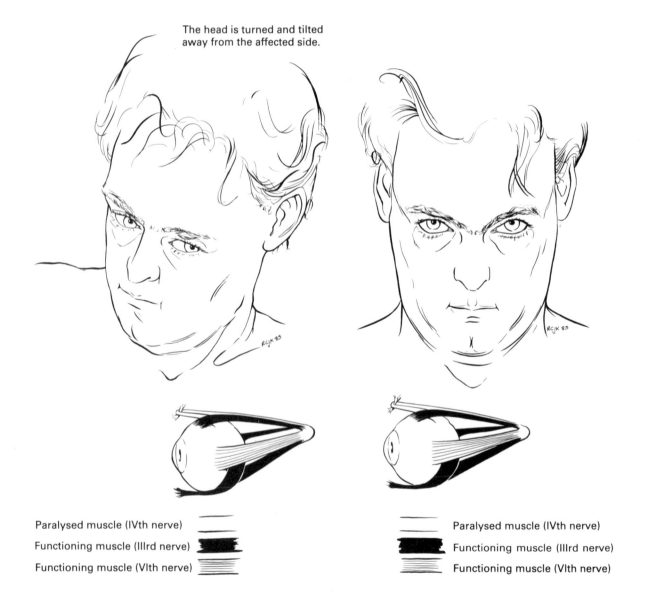

The head is turned and tilted away from the affected side.

Paralysed muscle (IVth nerve)

Functioning muscle (IIIrd nerve)

Functioning muscle (VIth nerve)

Paralysed muscle (IVth nerve)

Functioning muscle (IIIrd nerve)

Functioning muscle (VIth nerve)

c. Sixth nerve palsy
Unilateral:
This shows head turn to the affected side (Fig. 4.20).

Fig. 4.20 Unilateral VIth nerve palsy (left eye).

Unopposed medial rectus turns eye inwards.
Head moves to affected side to regain parallel gaze.

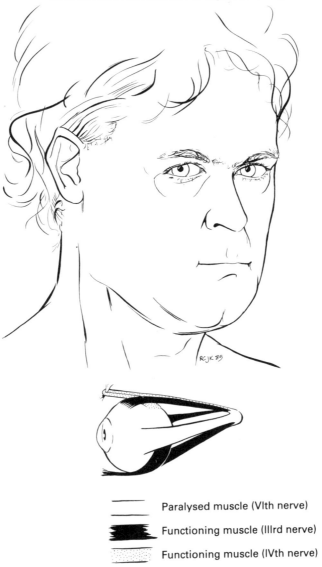

—— Paralysed muscle (VIth nerve)

███ Functioning muscle (IIIrd nerve)

▒▒▒ Functioning muscle (IVth nerve)

Bilateral:
This show no characteristic head posture, but:
– all distant images are doubled
– the patient can usually read without double vision.

Examination for squint and ocular muscle imbalance

Ask the patient to observe a distant object.

– Are the eyes straight?

If the eyes are straight, the reflections on each cornea should be symmetrical. Observe the patient from the same level, using the inspection torch (Fig. 4.21).

Confirm the observation by the cover/uncover test, using a small card.

THE COVER TEST

Note the corneal reflections. Are they:

– central?
– eccentric?

Cover the right eye, observing the left eye (Fig. 4.22). Did the left eye move:

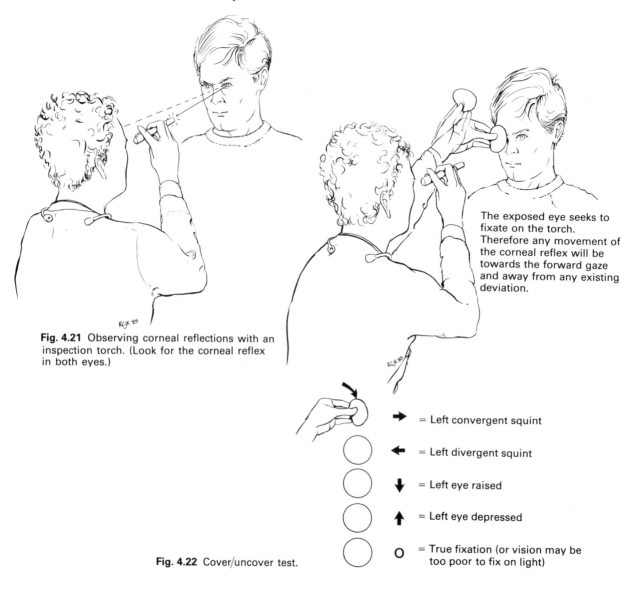

The exposed eye seeks to fixate on the torch. Therefore any movement of the corneal reflex will be towards the forward gaze and away from any existing deviation.

Fig. 4.21 Observing corneal reflections with an inspection torch. (Look for the corneal reflex in both eyes.)

➡ = Left convergent squint

⬅ = Left divergent squint

⬇ = Left eye raised

⬆ = Left eye depressed

O = True fixation (or vision may be too poor to fix on light)

Fig. 4.22 Cover/uncover test.

Direction of movement of exposed eye
- out? = left convergent squint
- in? = left divergent squint
- down? = left eye raised
- up? = left eye depressed
- combination = compound horizontal/vertical
- no movement = left eye fixing true, or vision is very poor and patient is unable to see the target

Repeat, covering the left eye and observing the right, because:
- there may be a deviation of the right eye
- an alternating deviation may be present

On removing the cover from the eye, observe it for movement.
- If it alone moves in any direction to take up fixation there is a latent deviation.
- If no movement is seen on performing all these tests, the ocular muscle balance is normal.

If a squint is demonstrated, cover the straight eye and observe the correcting movement of the squinting eye.

This movement can be seen more easily by alternate cover from one eye to the other, which will demonstrate a latent as well as a manifest squint and reveal the maximum angle of deviation.

If there is an abnormal head posture, the test should be repeated in the abnormal position to determine if the deviation is relieved or reduced.

Range of ocular movement
Ask the patient:
- to keep the head still
- to look at the light in your inspection torch, and
- to follow its movement.

Note the position of the lids. A slight unilateral ptosis may be associated with a superior rectus palsy. A gross ptosis may indicate a IIIrd nerve palsy.

Ocular movements are tested from the primary position to show if:
- each eye has a full range into all the directions of gaze (Fig. 4.23)
- double vision is noticed in any direction
- there is any nystagmoid jerking. This indicates:
  recovery of a paresis
  a cerebellar lesion.

a. IIIrd nerve
The eye is divergent, but can move outwards (VIth nerve, lateral rectus). There is a wheel rotation of the iris on attempting to look medially (IVth nerve, superior oblique). The pupil is dilated and fixed to light stimulus, but the other pupil reacts consensually.

b. IVth nerve
The eye drifts up when the patient looks medially. Torsion (wheel rotation of the eye) disorientates the image seen by the patient and causes some distress.

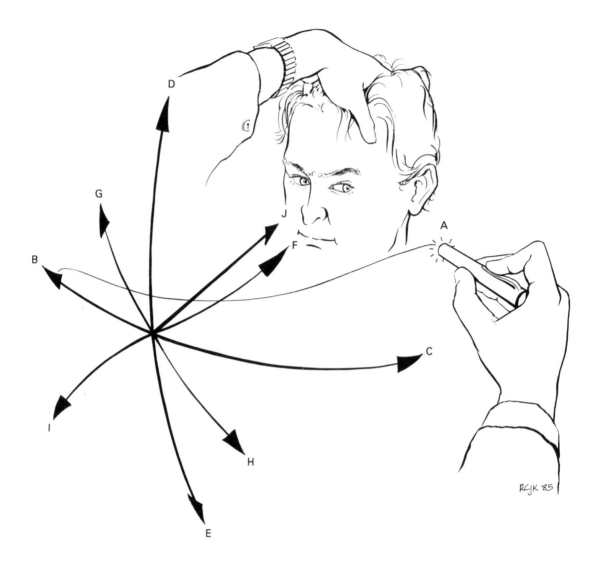

Fig. 4.23 Testing the range of ocular movement.

c. VIth nerve
The eye can reach the midline, but cannot turn out further.

Record your findings.

Ocular adnexae
It is unlikely that the adnexae will be injured in isolation, but bear in mind the possibility that they have been included in other local damage.

Lacerations of the lateral portion of the upper lid may involve the lacrimal gland (Fig. 4.24).

Injuries at the medial canthus (Fig. 4.25) may involve the lacrimal canaliculi and the lacrimal sac.

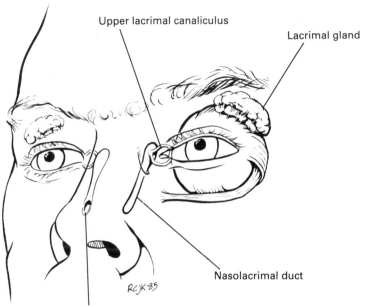

Fig. 4.24 Lacrimal apparatus.

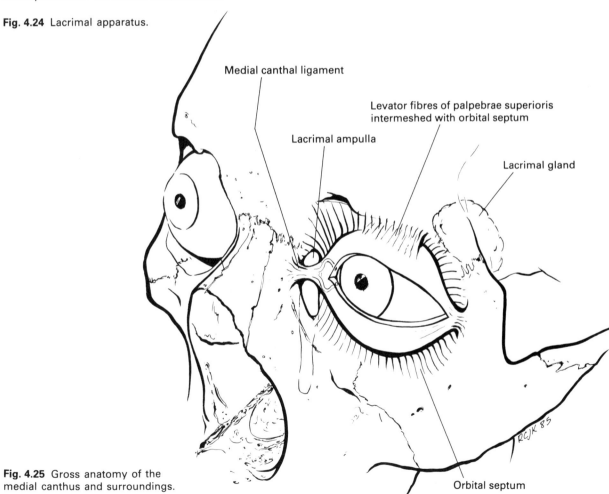

Fig. 4.25 Gross anatomy of the medial canthus and surroundings.

Hooks and dog bites pulling on the outer parts of the lids can:
– tear either lid through the canaliculus medially
– dislocate the medial canthal ligament (Fig. 4.26).

The upper canaliculus commonly remains intact.

Fig. 4.26 Canthal damage due to tugging injury of lid by dog bite, hook, etc.

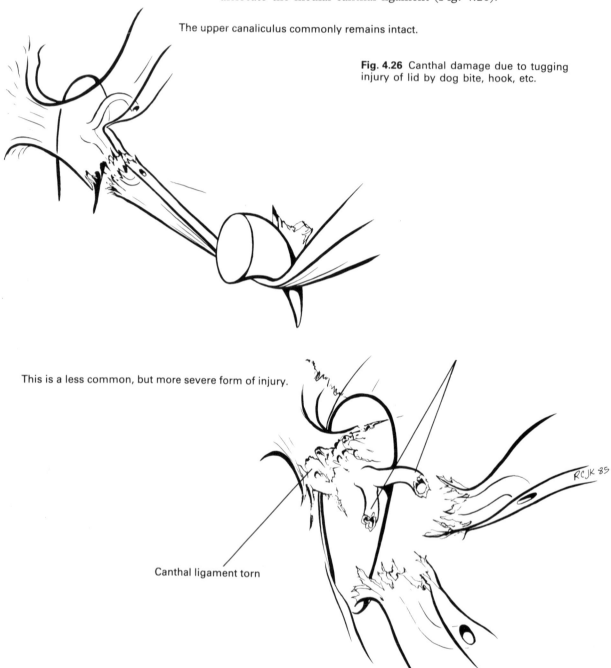

This is a less common, but more severe form of injury.

Canthal ligament torn

Lids

Extreme blepharospasm is seen with diffuse epithelial loss or damage in some burns and particularly with welding flash or other sudden u.v. light exposure (electrical short circuits). It also sometimes presents as an hysterical condition.

a. Observe if the lids are swollen. Trauma often causes almost instant swelling of the lids from oedema or haemorrhage. The eye is closed tightly, so examination is very difficult. Blood is contained by the orbital fascia and is thus prevented from reaching the cheek and upper lip, but it can track invisibly over the nasal bridge to the other orbit, simulating bilateral injury. (See Figure 4.27).

Fig. 4.27 Gross anatomy of the orbital septum.

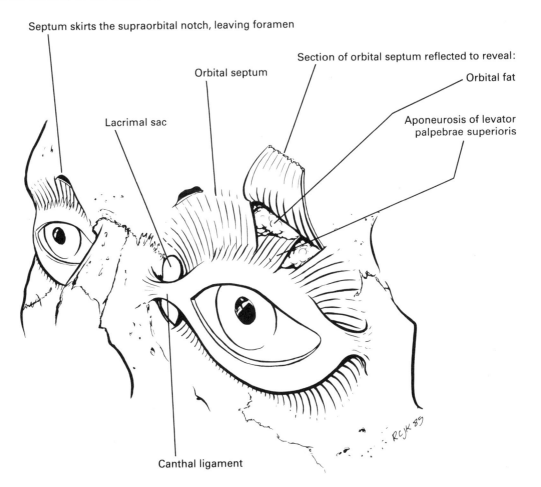

Septum skirts the supraorbital notch, leaving foramen

Section of orbital septum reflected to reveal:

Orbital septum

Orbital fat

Lacrimal sac

Aponeurosis of levator palpebrae superioris

Canthal ligament

When the swelling has subsided, there may be a residual drooping of the upper lid. This traumatic ptosis is commonly due to a dehiscence of the aponeurosis of the levator palpebrae and can occur after quite minor blunt injury (Fig. 4.28). The more remote possibility of an associated IIIrd nerve palsy must be excluded by confirming that the ocular movements and pupil reactions are normal.

b. If there is little or no swelling:
– are the orbits and lids bilaterally symmetrical?
– is the configuration of the lids normal? (Fig. 4.29).
– is there a laceration?

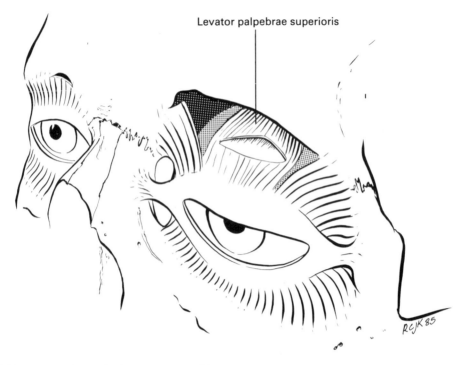

Levator palpebrae superioris

Fig. 4.28 Post-traumatic ptosis due to rupture of levator aponeurosis.

Fig. 4.29 Relation of lids, pupil and cornea in a normal eye.

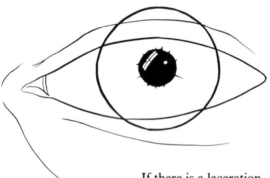

If there is a laceration, does it involve the lid margin? This will need careful reapposition using very fine instruments and materials. Does it involve the medial canthus?

There may be damage to the lacrimal puncta and canaliculae.

c. In thermal and chemical burns, ascertain if the lid margin is involved. If so, this can:

– damage and distort the eyelash follicles
– destroy the meibomiam ducts
– occlude the lacrimal canaliculi, with immediate
– irritation and lack of protection, and later
– aberrant lashes chronically irritating the eye
– intractable discomfort and overflow of tears

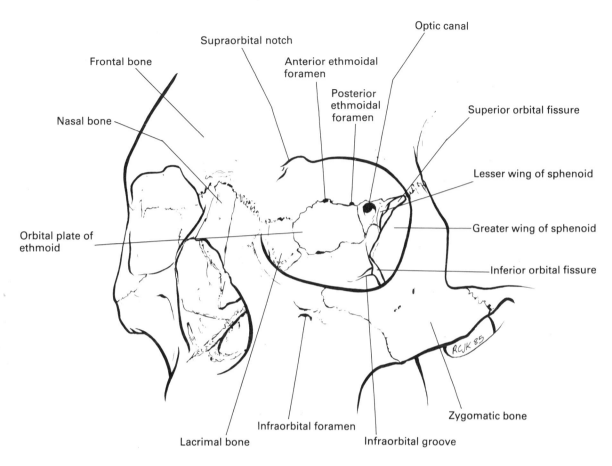

Fig. 4.30 The bony orbit.

Orbit (Fig. 4.30)

Orbital examination should follow after completion of the examination of the eyes and the central nervous system, having paid special attention to the size and reactions of the pupils, the sensation in the distribution of the trigeminal nerve (Fig. 4.31) (including the cornea) and the visual fields.

1. Consider:
– soft tissue damage
– possible introduction of foreign material (Fig. 4.32a)
Is there a fracture of the
– rim? (Fig. 4.32b)
– walls? (Fig. 4.32c)
– midface? (Figs. 4.32d, e, f, g)
– skull?
Is there associated damage to the:
– brain?
– visual pathways? (Fig. 4.32h)
– paranasal sinuses? (Fig. 4.32i)
– lacrimal gland? (Fig. 4.32j)
– lacrimal sac?
– nasolacrimal duct?

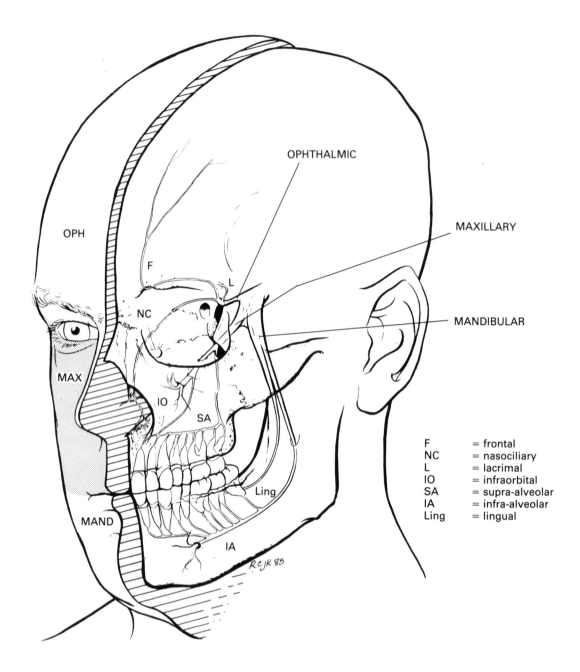

Fig. 4.31 The trigeminal nerve.

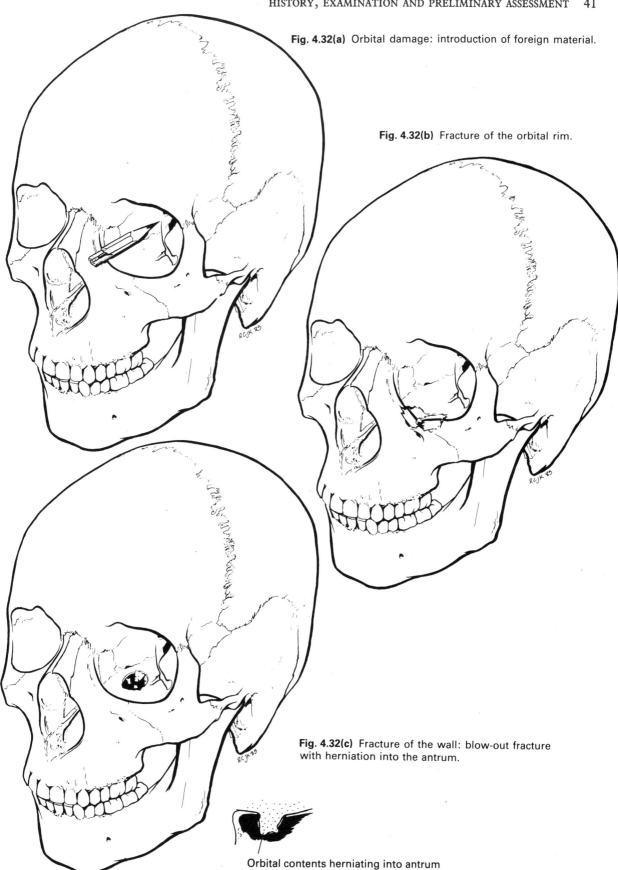

Fig. 4.32(a) Orbital damage: introduction of foreign material.

Fig. 4.32(b) Fracture of the orbital rim.

Fig. 4.32(c) Fracture of the wall: blow-out fracture with herniation into the antrum.

Orbital contents herniating into antrum

Fig. 4.32(d) Fractures of midface: Le Fort's fractures II and III.

Fig. 4.32(e) Zygomatic fracture.

Hinges here

Fig. 4.32(f) Complete zygomatic fracture.

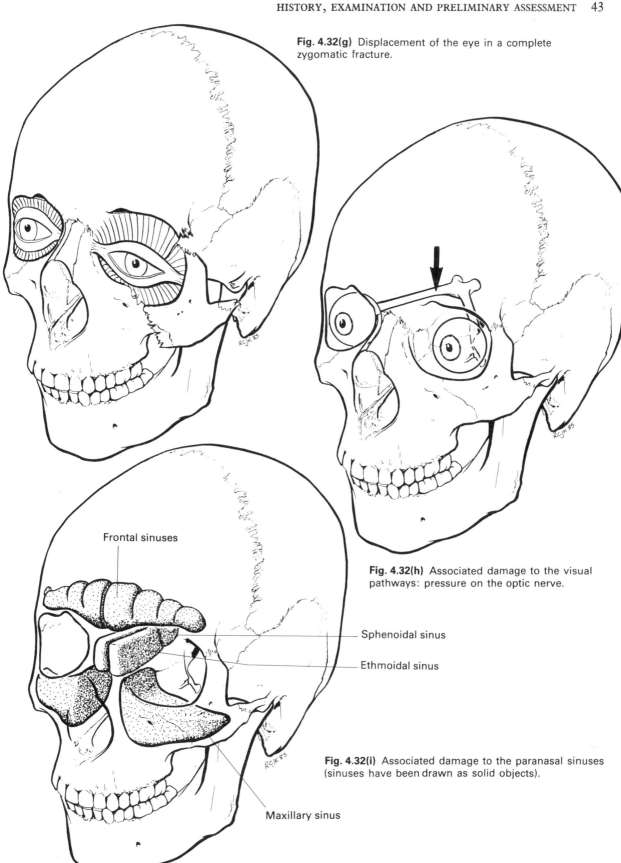

Fig. 4.32(g) Displacement of the eye in a complete zygomatic fracture.

Fig. 4.32(h) Associated damage to the visual pathways: pressure on the optic nerve.

Frontal sinuses

Sphenoidal sinus

Ethmoidal sinus

Fig. 4.32(i) Associated damage to the paranasal sinuses (sinuses have been drawn as solid objects).

Maxillary sinus

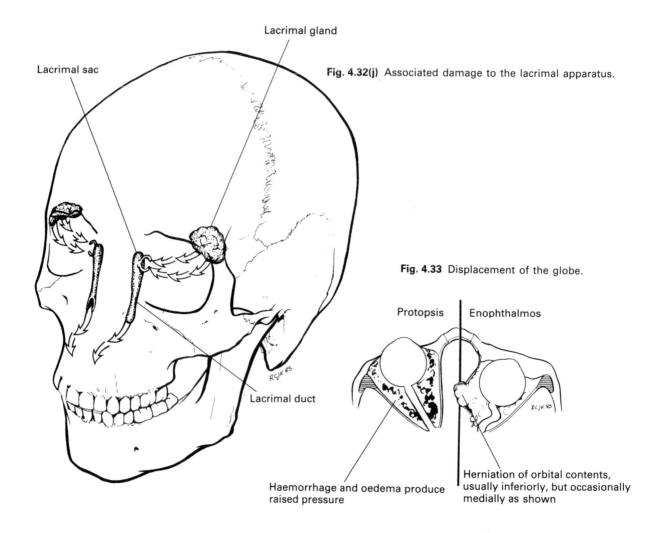

Lacrimal gland

Lacrimal sac

Fig. 4.32(j) Associated damage to the lacrimal apparatus.

Fig. 4.33 Displacement of the globe.

Protopsis

Enophthalmos

Lacrimal duct

Haemorrhage and oedema produce raised pressure

Herniation of orbital contents, usually inferiorly, but occasionally medially as shown

2. Look for:
– CSF leak: rhinorrhoea
– epistaxis
– pulsation in the orbit: frontal lobe prolapse, caroticocavernous fistula
– blindness from pressure on the optic nerve
– corneal exposure from displacement of the globe
– sub-conjunctival haemorrhage with no posterior limit

3. Are the bony walls of the orbit intact? If there is much oedema, this will be difficult to decide without an X-ray. It is easy to overlook a fracture, because of multiple injury, suffusion, shock and concussion.

4. Is the globe displaced? (Fig. 4.33.) This can be:
– proptosis due to haemorrhage and oedema
– enophthalmos due to fracture of the orbital walls and herniation of orbital contents

These may cancel out at first. The globe may also be displaced downwards or laterally.

There is sensory loss in the maxillary area if the orbital floor is fractured (Figs. 4.34a,b). X-ray including orbital tomography is needed for diagnosis.

5. Consider the danger of cellulitis.

6. Palpate the orbit. Is there:
– local tenderness?
– deformity (step defect of orbital rim)?
– loss of continuity (separation of fronto-zygomatic suture)?
– crepitation?

Surgical emphysema suggests a 'blow-out' fracture and there is a risk of infection.

7. Is there double vision? This may be due to:
– incarceration of muscle (Fig. 4.34c)
– laceration of muscle
– displacement of the trochlea
– nerve damage at muscle entry or orbital apex
– decompensation of a pre-existent squint

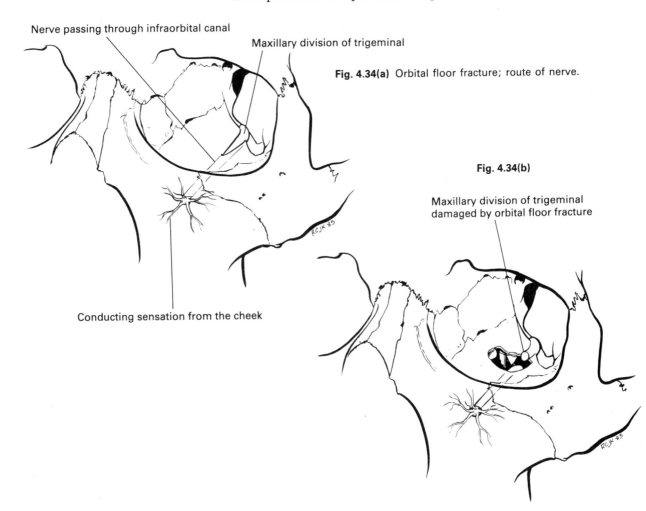

Nerve passing through infraorbital canal

Maxillary division of trigeminal

Fig. 4.34(a) Orbital floor fracture; route of nerve.

Fig. 4.34(b)

Maxillary division of trigeminal damaged by orbital floor fracture

Conducting sensation from the cheek

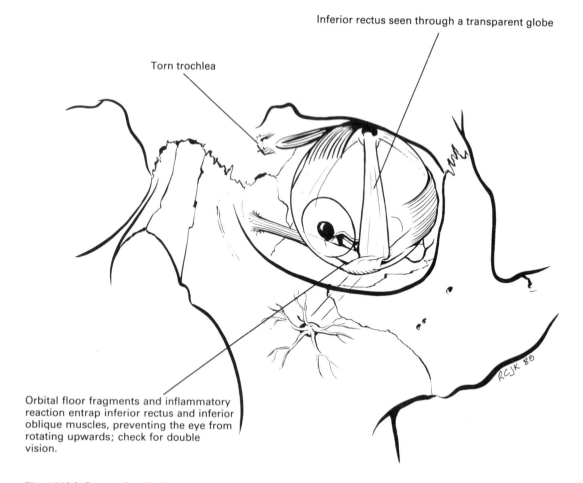

Inferior rectus seen through a transparent globe

Torn trochlea

Orbital floor fragments and inflammatory reaction entrap inferior rectus and inferior oblique muscles, preventing the eye from rotating upwards; check for double vision.

Fig. 4.34(c) Composite drawing showing trochlear damage and blow-out fracture (unlikely to be occasioned by the same injury).

ASSESSMENT

The history and examination findings may allow a firm conclusion on diagnosis and management. There are some features worthy of special mention.

Pain in the eye may be severe from superficial corneal damage, from spasm of the iris sphincter and from an acute rise of intraocular pressure. Surface pain may be caused by a concealed foreign body, typically held in the upper sub-tarsal groove, from which it can be removed after eversion of the lid. See Figures 4.35a, b, c and 4.36 and page 73.

Abrasion and laceration
A corneal abrasion is very painful and does not show well unless the surface is stained with sterile fluorescein, when it becomes very obvious (Fig. 4.37). Conjunctival lacerations are similarly well demonstrated by fluorescein.

Fig. 4.35 Eversion of the lid to remove a foreign body.

Fig. 4.36 Corneal abrasions.

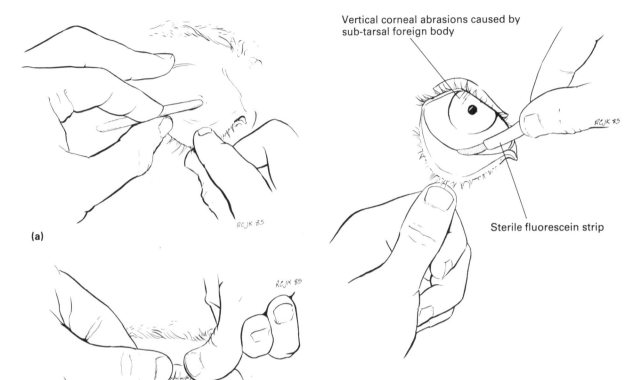

Vertical corneal abrasions caused by sub-tarsal foreign body

Sterile fluorescein strip

(a)

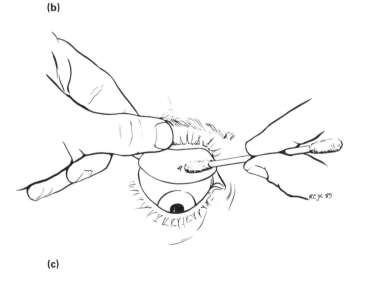

(b)

(c)

Fig. 4.37 Corneal and conjunctival abrasion.

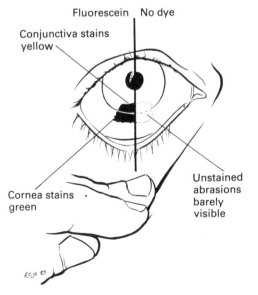

Fluorescein   No dye

Conjunctiva stains yellow

Cornea stains green

Unstained abrasions barely visible

Contact lenses of small diameter are worn much more frequently than larger ones, and there is an increasing number of attendances at ophthalmic and general A&E department for complications. Corneal oedema and abrasion are caused by overwearing, and patients may present in the early hours with pain, photophobia and blepharospasm from this cause.

When a lens drops out, it is difficult to find. Sometimes it is thought to have dropped out when in reality it has slipped into the upper fornix of the conjunctival sac where, after some time, it can produce a painful inflammatory reaction (Fig. 4.38).

Fig. 4.38 Contact lens in the upper fornix.

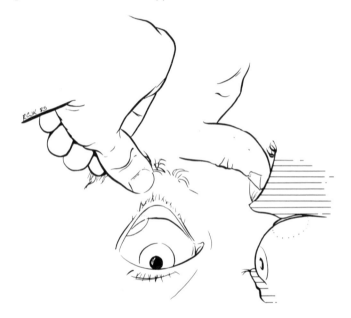

The most frequent use of contact lenses is for short-sight errors (myopia). Spectacle lenses for this condition are concave and are usually obviously thick-edged. Bear in mind that myopic eyes are more prone to vitreous and retinal problems.

Vitreous and retinal detachment
Sudden visual disturbance may be due to vitreous or retinal detachment, and very careful ophthalmoscopic examination is necessary. After an injury, a complaint of floaters usually means that the posterior segment of the eye (Fig. 4.39) is involved, and this should alert the examiner to the possibility of more serious damage than might at first appear. A complaint of seeing flashes of light means retinal damage and is almost certainly serious (Fig. 4.40a, b).

Although a small haemorrhage in the anterior chamber will usually absorb quickly without noticeable sequelae, an unpredictable proportion of patients will suffer secondary haemorrhage which is always more severe and may lead to serious complications. Therefore even a small hyphaema warrants referral to an ophthalmic unit.

Fig. 4.39 Gross anatomy of vitreous gel.

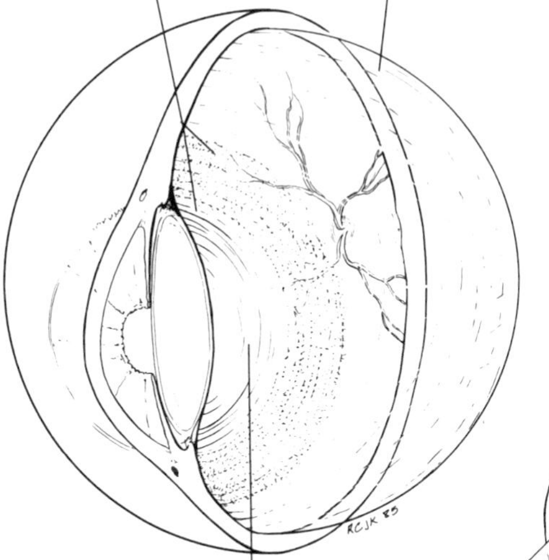

Vitreous attached in a band bridging the ora serrata (the vitreous base) and, less strongly, at the optic nerve head

Surface contact of vitreous to retina

Fig. 4.40(a) Traumatic vitreous detachment with retinal hole formation

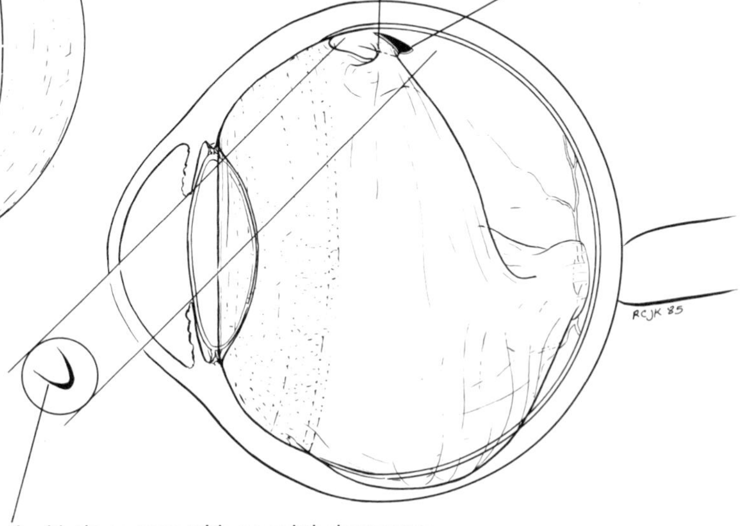

Vitreous tug stimulates the retina, causing flashing lights

Retinal hole

Anterior hyaloid face

Retinal hole as seen with an ophthalmoscope

Fig. 4.40(b) Traumatic retinal detachment.

Fluid penetrates the hole, detaching the whole retina from the underlying pigment layer

Piece of retina torn away

Vitreous base

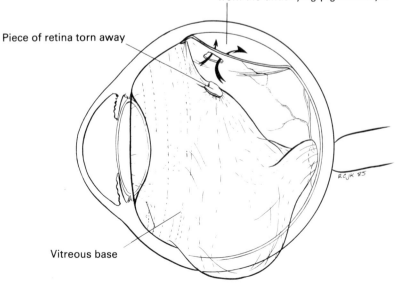

Blunt injury

Severe blunt injury can cause rupture and disorganisation of the eye. Even in injuries of lesser severity there is usually more than one area of damage in an organ as small as the eye.

Intraocular haemorrhage is frequent from tears of the uveal tissue and there may be cataract or dislocation of the lens and damage to the retina (Fig. 4.41).

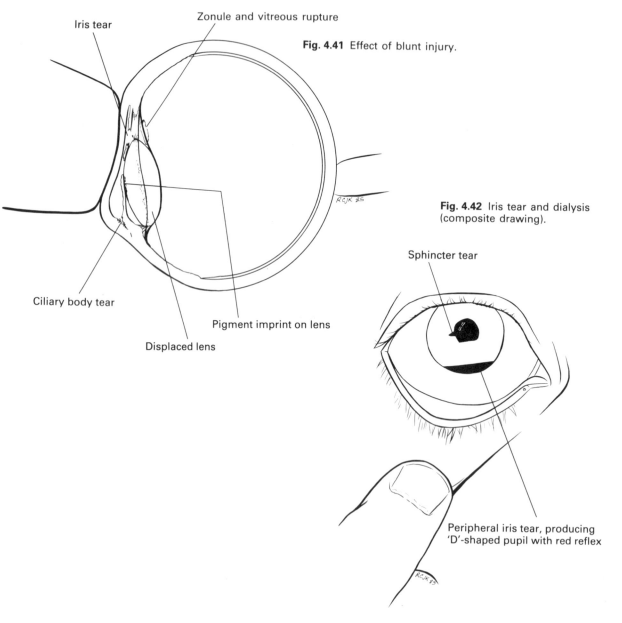

Iris tear

Zonule and vitreous rupture

Fig. 4.41 Effect of blunt injury.

Ciliary body tear

Displaced lens

Pigment imprint on lens

Fig. 4.42 Iris tear and dialysis (composite drawing).

Sphincter tear

Peripheral iris tear, producing 'D'-shaped pupil with red reflex

Iris tears are seen at the sphincter extending radially and showing well against the red reflex. The iris may also be torn at its root, causing a D-shaped pupil with a red reflex at the periphery (Fig. 4.42).

Pale crescent surrounded by blood

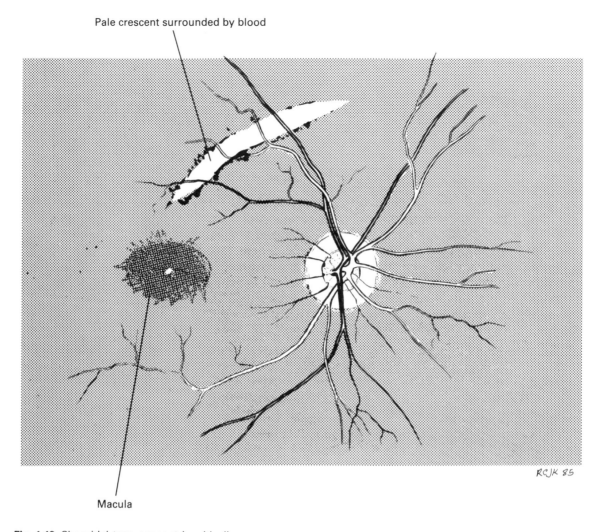

Macula

Fig. 4.43 Choroidal tear, concentric with disc.

Choroidal tears are concealed at an early stage by haemorrhage. They usually occur near to the optic disc (Fig. 4.43).

Concussion cataract often gives a radiating lace-like appearance against the red reflex when observing with an ophthalmoscope from a few inches away (Fig. 4.44).

The edge of a dislocated lens can often be seen within the pupil in the same manner, but with lesser displacement; it is indicated by a tremulous unsupported iris (Fig. 4.45).

Injury to the retina is shown by oedema which may be transient or prolonged; it shows as a cloudy white patch obscuring the underlying choroidal pattern. There may be tears at the site of oedema or at a previously compromised area of thinning or vitreoretinal adhesion. A tear shows up as red, because the choroid is seen through it, surrounded by grey detached retina. The short-sighted eye is more vulnerable.

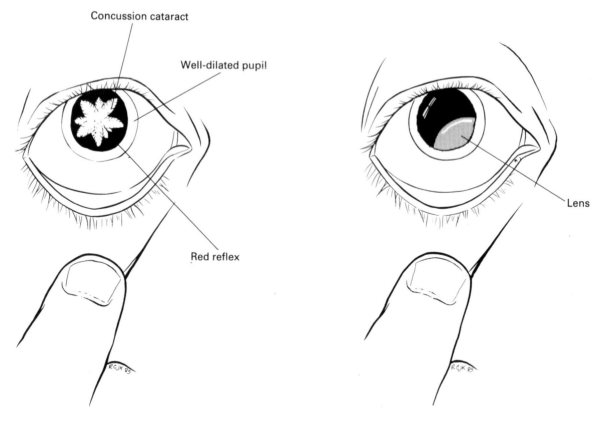

Fig. 4.44 Concussion cataract.

Fig. 4.45 Dislocated lens.

Perforating injury

Perforating injuries of the eye may not be obvious: small wounds of the cornea may be self-sealing and concealed against the background of the iris. Larger wounds are obvious: the eye has lost volume, the anterior chamber is absent or very shallow, the pupil distorted with prolapse of iris, and there may be swollen opaque lens matter protruding through a torn lens capsule. Wounds of the sclera are likely to be obscured by sub-conjunctival bleeding from superficial or deep vessels.

Lids

After considering conditions in which sight is threatened, injuries to the lids may seem trivial, but in the long term they may be very distressing to the patient.

If the inner angle is torn, the lacrimal drainage channels may be blocked, leading to intractable watering of the eye.

Inaccurate re-apposition of full-thickness lacerations at the lid margin leads not only to unsightly notching, but often to aberrant growth of eyelashes which can dangerously irritate the cornea. These wounds should be closed in three layers by ophthalmic plastic surgical methods with very fine sutures (Figs. 4.46a–e).

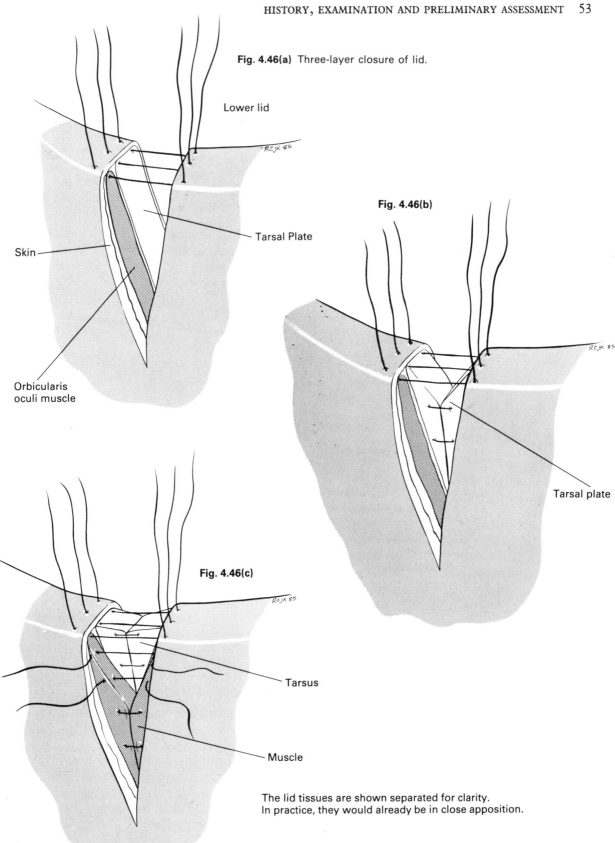

Fig. 4.46(a) Three-layer closure of lid.

Lower lid

Tarsal Plate

Skin

Orbicularis
oculi muscle

Fig. 4.46(b)

Tarsal plate

Fig. 4.46(c)

Tarsus

Muscle

The lid tissues are shown separated for clarity.
In practice, they would already be in close apposition.

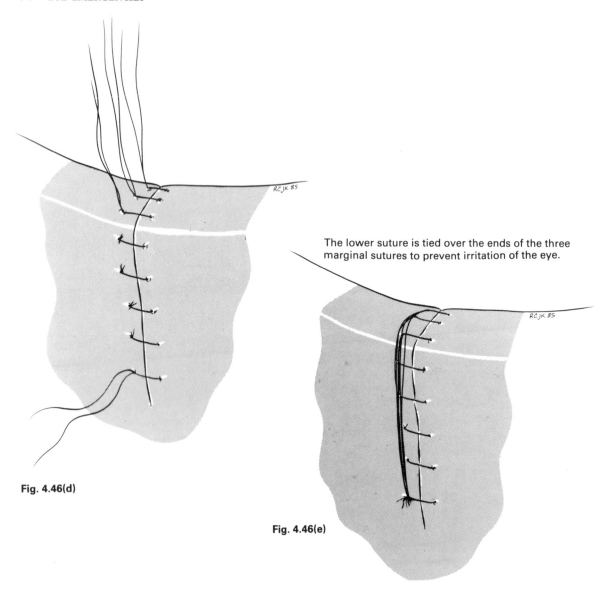

RC JK 85

The lower suture is tied over the ends of the three
marginal sutures to prevent irritation of the eye.

RC JK 85

Fig. 4.46(d)

Fig. 4.46(e)

In full-thickness injuries of the upper lid, the levator aponeurosis
may be damaged, resulting in ptosis. In fact, the aponeurosis is so
delicate it can be torn by minor blunt injury.

Orbit

In the early period after orbital injury, swelling may conceal the presence of a fracture of either the margin or orbital wall. Haematoma will
restrict movement, and it is very difficult to determine if there is
muscle incarceration in a 'blow-out' fracture line (Fig. 4.47).

It has been the fashion to repair such cases early, but conservative
management has shown that function is recovered spontaneously in
most cases. The casualty officer should be aware of the possibilities
and alert the ophthalmic and maxillofacial units at an early stage so
that the correct management can be planned.

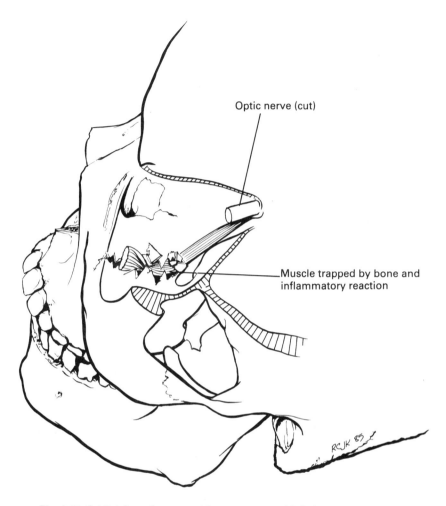

Optic nerve (cut)

Muscle trapped by bone and inflammatory reaction

Fig. 4.47 Orbital floor fracture with entrapment of inferior rectus.

NON-TRAUMATIC CASES

HISTORY

Take the history, recording:
- the presenting symptom (see Flow Diagram 3.1, page 9).
- its duration
- additional symptoms, both ophthalmic and systemic
- their duration

Refer to Flow Diagrams 3.2 and 3.3 (pages 11, 15) if the patient presents with an acute red eye, after observing the distribution of the redness. Acute iritis and acute glaucoma are the most serious ocular conditions. Caroticocavernous fistula and cavernous sinus thrombosis are serious systemic causes of a red eye, but are now rare.

Flow Diagrams 3.4 and 3.6 (pages 16 and 17) also give guidance on the causes of ocular pain and loss of vision. These include a number of conditions which seriously threaten vision. The more urgent again include acute glaucoma and acute iritis.

Among the conditions without ocular pain, giant cell arteritis, retinal detachment, central retinal arterial occlusion and intracranial aneurysm may require urgent action. See Flow Diagram 3.5 (page 17).

In these and other more obscure cases a more complete history is needed:
- Is there some old or more recent event leading up to the emergency presentation?
- Is there a general medical condition which could predispose to the presenting ocular problem?

EXAMINATION

The patient is made comfortable, lying down or sitting with the head supported.

Equipment required (see also page 68):
- an inspection torch
- an ophthalmoscope

1. Check the visual acuity.

Check one eye at a time, covering the other with a card or the palm of the hand (not with the fingers, because it may be possible to see through a gap between them).

The visual acuity can be checked first on the distance test chart, and only if the patient cannot see the top letter are the poorer levels of acuity tested.

2. Check the pupil reactions.

The pupil reactions can give much useful information on both sensory and motor lesions. When there is sensory loss, alternate stimulation of each eye may show an unexpected, paradoxical, dilatation of the pupil of the impaired eye as the light is shone on it,

Flow Diagram 4.1

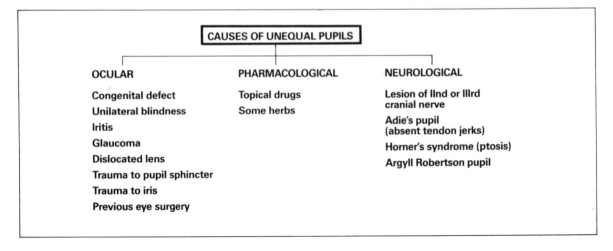

CAUSES OF UNEQUAL PUPILS		
OCULAR	**PHARMACOLOGICAL**	**NEUROLOGICAL**
Congenital defect	Topical drugs	Lesion of IInd or IIIrd cranial nerve
Unilateral blindness	Some herbs	Adie's pupil (absent tendon jerks)
Iritis		Horner's syndrome (ptosis)
Glaucoma		Argyll Robertson pupil
Dislocated lens		
Trauma to pupil sphincter		
Trauma to iris		
Previous eye surgery		

because the residual consensual constriction is stronger than that to direct light. This is an afferent defect of pupil reaction and is a delicate test for use in doubtful cases (Fig. 4.48).

3. Test the visual field of each eye separately.

Fig. 4.48 Scheme of afferent pupil defect.

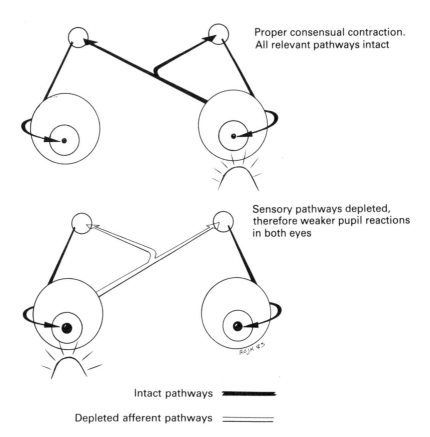

Proper consensual contraction. All relevant pathways intact

Sensory pathways depleted, therefore weaker pupil reactions in both eyes

Intact pathways

Depleted afferent pathways

The visual fields will need assessment by confrontation. In ocular conditions this may not be easy, because of a gentle gradation. A small white spherical target should be used for the test. The patient is asked to fix his/her gaze on the examiner's pupil, so the examiner can observe that fixation is maintained during the examination. The target is brought into the field from the periphery and the patient asked to indicate when it is first seen. The examiner can then compare the patient's field with his/her own. See Figures 4.49 and 4.50.

In most defects of the visual pathways the loss is sharply demarcated (Fig. 4.51) and can be demonstrated to a moving finger or the end of a cotton bud.

Field defects may not be peripheral. Central defects or distortions can be shown by the patient's observation of a grid pattern, particularly a white grid on a black background (Amsler's Chart) (Fig. 4.52).

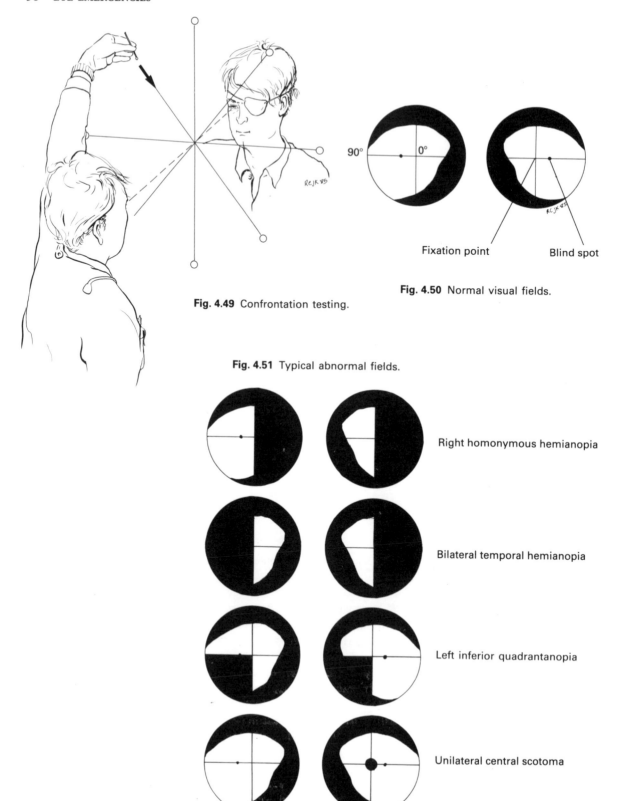

Fig. 4.49 Confrontation testing.

90°   0°

Fixation point   Blind spot

Fig. 4.50 Normal visual fields.

Fig. 4.51 Typical abnormal fields.

Right homonymous hemianopia

Bilateral temporal hemianopia

Left inferior quadrantanopia

Unilateral central scotoma

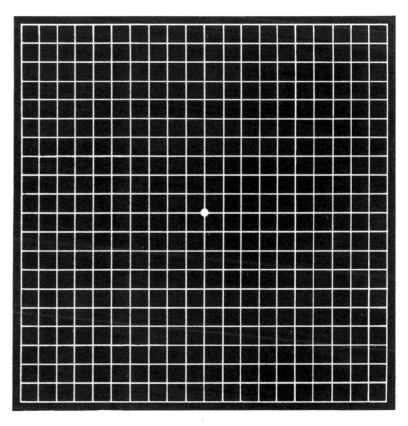

Fig. 4.52 Amsler's chart. (Reproduced with kind permission from Hamblin Instruments.)

Hemianopic defects due to cortical lesions, and bitemporal defects, may easily be missed because patients are not fully aware of them. A sudden and complete bitemporal hemianopia suggests infarction of a chromophobe adenoma of the pituitary gland (pituitary apoplexy).

Interpretation of subjective tests of visual acuity and fields
It is important to remember that the usual tests of visual acuity and field are subjective and depend for accuracy not only on the examiner, but on the patient. Anxiety, hysteria or malingering will give false results. Patients with such problems are very likely to present themselves first in an A&E department. If the examiner is misled, symptoms can be further exaggerated and subsequent evaluation and management made more difficult. Several such patients will have been subjected to invasive investigations before the non-organic nature of their presentation is finally established.

In a visual acuity test the genuine ophthalmic patient will read the chart quite quickly and begin to make mistakes on difficult letters

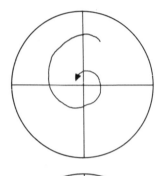

before giving up. Non-genuine reading is usually painfully slow and deliberate, with a sharp cut-off at the chosen level of amblyopia, but no mistakes.

Patients with hysterical blindness can usually ambulate safely, although denying light perception. The blink reflex to menace is usually present and the pupil reactions are normal. Charting of field defects shows bizarre and nonsensical results, such as spiral contraction, crossed isoptres, stellate defects, tubular fields and smaller fields to larger objects when the test is first made with smaller objects (Fig. 4.53)

Fig. 4.53 Bizzare fields in hysterical blindness.

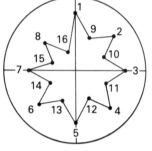

Numbers indicate the sequence of testing.

1st object

2nd, smaller object

3rd, large object

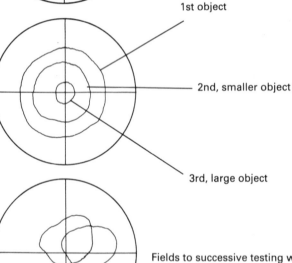

Fields to successive testing with similar objects

Patients will have normal optokinetic nystagmus which can be demonstrated by slow rotation of a drum with black and white vertical lines held closely before the eyes (optokinetic drum). Visually evoked cortical responses are normal (Fig. 4.54).

Visual fields can show characteristic non-organic changes on formal testing by perimetry, but confrontation testing is usually an 'all-or-none' response.

The remainder of the examination follows a sequence of inspection of the anterior followed by the posterior structures of the eye, using good illumination and an inspection torch.

4. Inspect the face:
– Is the lid configuration normal?
– Are the lid apertures equal?

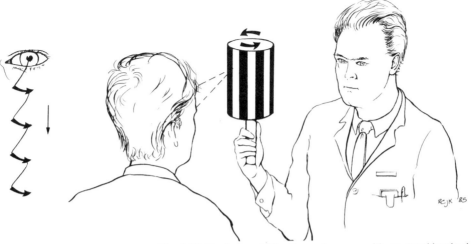

Fig. 4.54 Testing optokinetic nystagmus with an optokinetic drum.

— Is the appearance of the lid margins normal?

Spastic entropion may present with symptoms of a superficial foreign body in the eye. The lashes are rolled in and hidden from view until the lid skin is pulled down towards the orbital margin.

— Is one eye more prominent than the other?
— Is there swelling? If so:
— Is it due to oedema or inflammation?
— Is it generalised or localised?

Inflammatory conditions of the lids, adnexae and orbit may present as emergencies. They will show the usual signs of inflammation localised to the area concerned and will include orbital oedema, orbital cellulitis, acute infection of the lacrimal gland (dacryoadenitis) and lacrimal sac (dacryocystitis) (Fig. 4.55).

Fig. 4.55 Acute dacryocystitis.

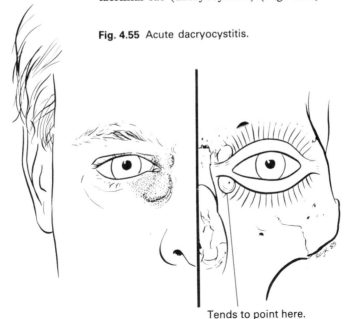

Tends to point here.

5. Inspect the conjunctiva and sclera:
– Is the appearance normal?

Look at the vascular pattern and the number of visible blood vessels:
– Are the blood vessels injected? If so:
– Is this inflammatory or congestive?
– What is the distribution of vascular engorgement?

In conjunctivitis the conjunctiva generally shows an overall flush. In episcleritis and scleritis there is localised inflammation. In keratitis, iritis, cyclitis and acute glaucoma there is limbal and circumcorneal injection (Fig. 4.56)

– Is there localised swelling? This suggests inflammation (episcleritis, scleritis, foreign body reaction).

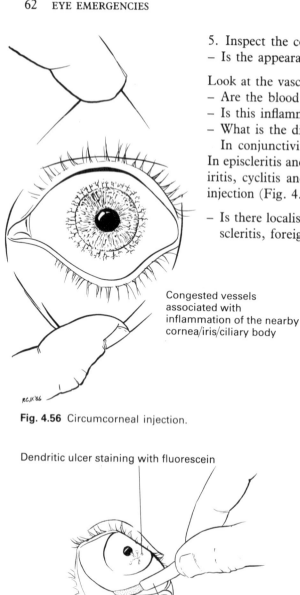

Congested vessels associated with inflammation of the nearby cornea/iris/ciliary body

Fig. 4.56 Circumcorneal injection.

Dendritic ulcer staining with fluorescein

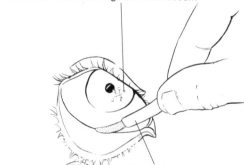

Sterile fluorescein strip

Fig. 4.57 Estimating intraocular pressure.

6. Estimate the intraocular pressure, with the patient looking downwards, by palpating the globe gently through the upper lid (above the tarsal cartilage where it is thinner) using both forefingers on each eye in turn. The other fingers should be supported on the brow to ensure better control (Fig. 4.57).

7. Inspect the cornea:
– Is it brightly reflecting and transparent?

An active lesion causing an opacity will have related local vascular injection at the limbus and may stain with fluorescein. In its early stages herpes simplex (dendritic ulcer) does not show as an opacity, but it will stain (Fig. 4.58).

Fig. 4.58 Herpes simplex.

A steamy cornea is seen in acute glaucoma. Look for the other signs (Fig. 4.59). See page 81.

An acute swelling and dense cloudy opacity (acute hydrops) can occur in advanced conical cornea. This is rare but dramatic, and probably follows a bout of rubbing.

– Are there cellular deposits on the back of the cornea? This is an indication of iridocyclitis (keratic precipitates) (Fig. 4.60).

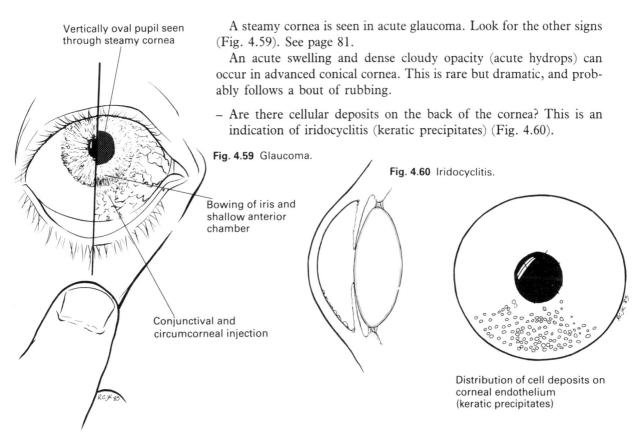

Vertically oval pupil seen through steamy cornea

Bowing of iris and shallow anterior chamber

Conjunctival and circumcorneal injection

Fig. 4.59 Glaucoma.

Fig. 4.60 Iridocyclitis.

Distribution of cell deposits on corneal endothelium (keratic precipitates)

8. Look into the anterior chamber:
– Does it contain clear aqueous fluid? Turbidity obscures the iris details (iritis) (Fig. 4.61).

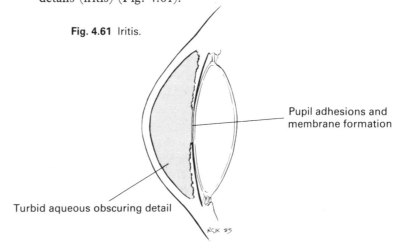

Fig. 4.61 Iritis.

Pupil adhesions and membrane formation

Turbid aqueous obscuring detail

– What is the pupil size?
– Is it the same in the two eyes? If unequal:
– Which is the abnormal pupil? The pupil is small in e.g.
iritis
convergence spasm (bilateral)

Horner's syndrome
brainstem lesions (bilateral)
and is enlarged in e.g.
IIIrd nerve palsy
acute glaucoma
severe visual loss
accidental contact with a mydriatic
- Is the iris pattern and colour normal? It is muddy and discoloured in acute iritis (Fig. 4.62).

Fig. 4.62 Acute iritis.

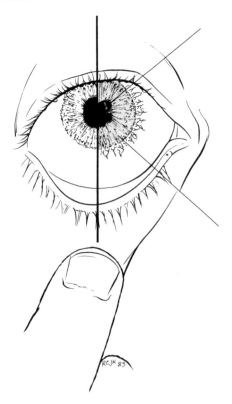

9. Look within the pupil, using the inspection torch:
- Are there any opacities to be seen? There could be inflammatory exudate in acute iritis. Cataract has a greyish-white appearance, but the lens in old persons can seem opaque until examined with the ophthalmoscope, when it is found to permit an easy view of the fundus.
10. Now examine with the ophthalmoscope from 20-30 cm:
- Is there a good red reflex? It can be impaired by:
corneal opacity
aqueous turbidity
pupillary exudate
lens opacity (cataract)
vitreous opacity
vitreous haemorrhage

The opacity can be localised by using parallax in relation to the pupil plane. If it is in front of the pupil, the opacity will move against the movement of the ophthalmoscope; if it is behind, it will move in the same direction (Fig. 4.63).

Fig. 4.63 Using parallax to locate intraocular features.

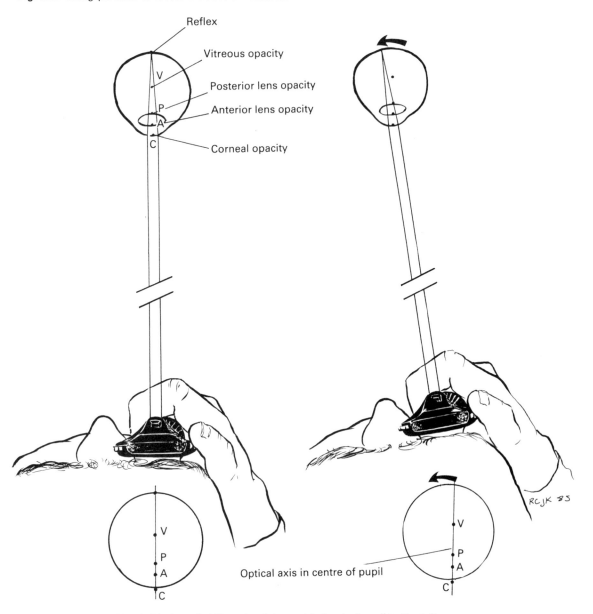

Reflex

Vitreous opacity

Posterior lens opacity

Anterior lens opacity

Corneal opacity

Optical axis in centre of pupil

Observer sees opacities behind pupil shift to the right, and in front of pupil to the left.

11. Approach more closely, still observing through the pupil and focus the ophthalmoscope.

The fundi are examined with special attention to the likely reasons for emergency presentation (see pages 16, 17). In many cases it will be helpful to dilate the pupil with a short-acting mydriatic (e.g. tropicamide 0.5%), so that the examination of the fundus is easier. In older patients without dilatation only the optic disc will be seen reasonably well, because the older the patient the smaller the pupil. The macula is particularly difficult to see because stimulation of that area by the light will cause further constriction.

Beware of the possibility of mydriasis (pupil dilatation) precipitating an acute glaucoma in older patients with:
– a history suggestive of glaucoma
– previous ocular surgery
– shallow anterior chambers

The presence of a shallow anterior chamber can be determined in this manner: If light is shone from the temporal side along the plane of the iris and the nasal side of the iris is in shadow, there is some shallowing.

Remember that the size and reactions of the pupils are important in the management of the unconscious patient and avoid the use of mydriatics in such cases.

Observe: optic disc, vessels, general background and then the macula.

a. Optic disc:
– colour, calibre of vessels, pressure on the globe required to cause pulsation
– Is there swelling or cupping?
b. Vessels:
– arteriovenous ratio, calibre, regularity, arteriovenous crossings
c. General background:
– haemorrhages, cytoid bodies (cotton wool spots), exudates
d. Macula
– oedema, haemorrhage
Repeat the procedure with the other eye.

Ocular movements
Ocular movements are checked with consideration of the possibility of IIIrd, IVth or VIth nerve involvement as a cause of double vision. (Refer to pages 27, 34). Convergence spasm may present as an emergency and may be mistaken for a bilateral VIth nerve palsy; but the spasm is associated with constricted pupils, which should alert the examiner to the true diagnosis.

ASSESSMENT

Prompt referral is needed in some cases.
There should be prompt referral is any case of:
– unexplained loss of vision, red eye or pain
– suspected acute glaucoma
– retinal detachment
– optic disc oedema with visual loss
– acute inflammation which threatens vision

In central retinal arterial obstruction, before referring, try:
- massage of the eye
- rebreathing to raise carbon dioxide level for vasodilatation

In all cases of transient loss of vision (amaurosis fugax) check for:
- hypertension
- blood dyscrasia
- heart disease
- carotid occlusion
- vertebrobasilar insufficiency
- Giant cell arteritis (ESR needed)

There should be prompt referral in any case of unexplained loss of vision, red eye or pain. The combination of these is a threat of permanent blindness. A painful red eye is a threat to sight even without loss of vision at presentation.

Circumcorneal injection indicates:
- keratitis
- acute iritis
- acute glaucoma

True rainbow haloes indicate a closed angle and the risk of acute glaucoma. Avoid asking a leading question. The other signs are listed on page 81, but their absence should not deter referral.

Retinal detachment

This diagnosis is suggested by a history of blurred vision preceded by an awareness of floating spots (vitreous disturbance) and peripheral flashes of light (retinal traction). A field defect is often unnoticed until the retina is detached close to or involving the macula (Fig. 4.64).

Fig. 4.64 Retinal detachment.

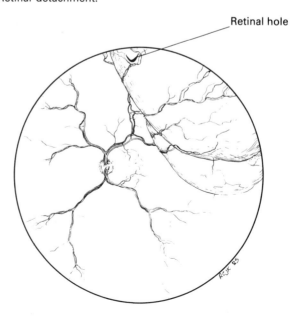

Retinal hole

After a tear the retina may be pulled or floated off as a grey membrane, losing the red appearance the transparent undetached retina is given by the choroid.

Using the ophthalmoscope held at a distance of about 30 cm from the eye, the red or grey reflex may be used to indicate the extent of detachment. A focused examination of the fundus will show the detail. This may need a dilated pupil.

It is possible to make a diagnosis of retinal detachment, even when corneal scarring or cataract prevent direct examination, by ultrasonography or computerised tomography (CT) scan.

Optic disc oedema with visual loss
This could be:
– chronic papilloedema with early consecutive optic atrophy. (Children are in greater danger of blindness from consecutive atrophy than adults.)
– papilloedema with optic nerve or chiasmal compression
– optic neuritis (Multiple sclerosis)
– ischaemic optic neuropathy (Giant cell arteritis)

Acute inflammations which threaten vision
These include:
– acute iritis
– ophthalmia neonatorum
– orbital cellulitis
– cavernous sinus thrombosis

Less urgent referrals are needed in cases of:
– excessive optic disc cupping (chronic glaucoma)
– asymmetrical optic disc cupping (chronic glaucoma)
– unequal pupil size or reactions without other signs (there are many possibilities)
Other conditions can probably be managed without referral unless they are persistent.

EXAMINATION OF THE EYE UNDER MAGNIFICATION

The key to successful recognition of clinical signs when examining the eyes is the use of magnification and good illumination. The larger A&E departments and any units receiving a significant number of ophthalmic emergencies need more specialised equipment than that described in the early parts of this chapter.

A modern slit-lamp microscope is invaluable for examination of the anterior segment of the eye. It produces a binocular erect image at chosen magnification and has integrated illumination of the point of examination. Its position can be adjusted with one hand so that detailed examination can be completed with speed and accuracy.

Many conditions which could otherwise pass unnoticed can easily be seen with the microscope, for example small superficial foreign bodies, penetrating wounds from objects of minute size, the track of intraocular foreign bodies with dimensions of less than 0.25 mm, flare in the anterior chamber and small abnormalities of the iris.

The removal of corneal foreign bodies is best performed on the slit-lamp microscope.

The slit-lamp can also be used for more specialised examinations of the intraocular pressure, the angle of the anterior chamber, the crystalline lens and for examination of the fundus.

The instrument will be of value to permanent staff in the A&E department and essential to any ophthalmic staff who are required to examine a patient in that department.

5

Diagnosis and management

MINOR CONDITIONS

Bruises, abrasions and lacerations
Superficial foreign bodies
Superficial burns
Conjunctivitis
Blepharitis
Contact dermatitis
Episcleritis

SERIOUS CONDITIONS (see page 78)

Acute ocular inflammation
Herpes zoster ophthalmicus
Swelling and inflammation of periocular tissues and orbit
More extensive and deeper burns
All chemical burns
Blunt and perforating injuries
Optic nerve damage
Orbital fractures
Rapid visual loss

MINOR CONDITIONS

BRUISES

Bruises of the lids require no more than simple management with a
supporting dressing, sometimes more comforting as a cold compress.
It is important to avoid missing more serious injury, which should be
suspected if there is a causal history of
– strong forces
– a heavy object, or
– high speed, and if there is
– lid oedema
– blood or pigment between the lids
– pupil irregularity
– blood in the anterior chamber

SUB-CONJUNCTIVAL HAEMORRHAGE

There is sudden onset without pain. It has a dramatic appearance, but is not serious in itself.
1. Find the posterior limit. If there is none, consider orbital fracture.
2. Check urine and blood pressure.
3. Reassure the patient. No treatment is needed.

ABRASIONS AND LACERATIONS

Scratches are usually made by objects such as a fingernail, branch, contact lens, etc. There is sharp stabbing pain, aggravated by movement and opening the eye. Healing is by epithelial slide and later by mitosis. A total abrasion is usually healed within 3–4 days.

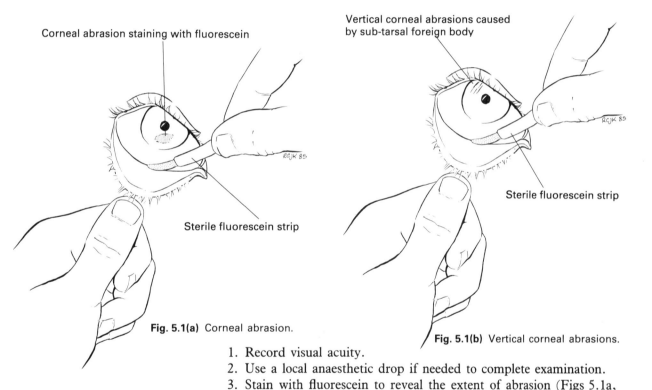

Fig. 5.1(a) Corneal abrasion.

Fig. 5.1(b) Vertical corneal abrasions.

1. Record visual acuity.
2. Use a local anaesthetic drop if needed to complete examination.
3. Stain with fluorescein to reveal the extent of abrasion (Figs 5.1a, b).
4. Check for a sub-tarsal foreign body.

Treatment
1. Avoid eye ointments or oily drops, which may impair healing.
2. Instil antibacterial eye drops for prophylaxis; instil mydriatic/cycloplegic to prevent pupil spasm.
3. Apply pad and bandage.
4. Refer cases if abrasion or laceration is extensive; review others in 24 hours.

RECURRENT ABRASIONS

These can occur for months or years after an earlier abrasion. Symptoms are typically most severe on waking.

Treatment
This is similar to above, but all such cases should be referred to an ophthalmologist. It may be necessary to use surgical toilet on the affected area to promote firm healing of epithelium to basement membrane.

CONJUNCTIVAL LACERATIONS

These are associated with sub-conjunctival haemorrhage. Stain with fluorescein.

Treatment
1. Topical antibiotic.
2. If the lacerations are extensive, bring them together with 8/0 or finer sutures.

LIDS

All lacerations near the medial canthus need to be checked for canalicular damage and damage to the medial canthal ligament. Reapposition needs to be prompt but accurate, using finer materials and instruments than are usually available in a general A&E department. Otherwise discomfort, watering, aberrant eyelashes and cosmetic deformity commonly result. It is usually better to refer without suture, because so often early attempts at repair have to be released and resutured to prevent deformity.

Secondary repair can be complicated.

NASOLACRIMAL DUCT

This is commonly lacerated in the following ways:
1. Damaged in medial wall orbital fracture
2. Torn canaliculus in hook or bite injury
3. Cicatrix of canaliculus after injury or burn

Treat later by dacryocystorhinostomy (DCR) after fractures.

SUPERFICIAL FOREIGN BODIES

Typically these cause sudden irritation in dust or wind. They produce surface pain, photophobia, grittiness on blinking.

CONJUNCTIVAL FOREIGN BODIES

1. Remove loose surface foreign bodies by irrigation or on a cotton bud.

2. Use fluorescein, because abrasion feels like a foreign body.
3. Check under the upper lid by eversion (Fig. 5.2a, b, c).

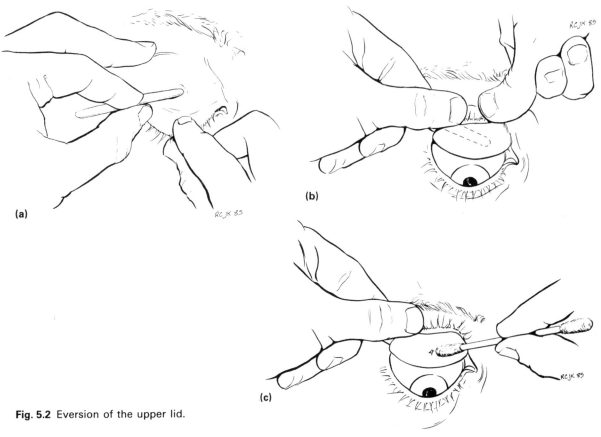

(a)

(b)

(c)

Fig. 5.2 Eversion of the upper lid.

Treatment
1. Remove embedded particles with a cotton bud or non-toothed fine forceps, after topical anaesthesia.
2. Give a topical antibiotic.
3. Apply a temporary eye pad for comfort.

SUBTARSAL FOREIGN BODIES

These arise from the same causes as superficial foreign bodies. There is more discomfort on blinking. Linear scratch marks show with fluorescein on upper cornea (Fig. 5.1b).

To extract, evert the upper lid. This is easy with practice.

Method for everting upper lid
1. Support the patient's head.
2. Instruct the patient to keep the eyes open and look down.
3. Hold the upper lid lashes between finger and thumb (Fig. 5.2a).
4. Place a matchstick, paperclip or a finger of the other hand on the upper lid just above the upper border of the tarsal plate.
5. Press down and back at this point (Fig. 5.2b).

Treatment
1. Remove the foreign body with a cotton bud (Fig. 5.2c).
2. Give a topical antibiotic.

CORNEAL FOREIGN BODIES

These are signalled by discomfort, often felt under the upper lid. You should suspect the possibility of a penetrating injury. Always confirm the history: Was a hammer being used? X-ray if in doubt.

Treatment
1. Instil topical anaesthetic.
2. Irrigate off with sterile fluid through a lacrimal cannula on a 2 ml syringe.
3. Avoid abrading with a cotton bud.
4. If the foreign body is embedded, refer the patient unless you are already practised in the use of a sterile needle or spud. Proper binocular magnification must be used.
5. Use fluorescein to indicate the extent of epithelial damage and record this on a diagram.
6. Instil antibacterial eye drops as prophylactic; instil mydriatic/cycloplegic to prevent pupil spasm.
7. Apply pad and bandage.
8. Review in 24 hours and refer the patient if the eye is red or uncomfortable.
9. Watch for infection.
10. Always refer a deeply embedded foreign body.

CONTACT LENS PROBLEMS

The most common problems are that the patient cannot remove the lens or the lens has become dislodged.
1. Ask the patient if the lens is soft or hard. If soft, the lens is difficult to see; refer to ophthalmologist or contact lens practitioner.
2. If hard, instil a topical anaesthetic.
3. Lift the upper lid towards the orbital rim and examine the upper conjunctival cul-de-sac (Fig. 5.3).

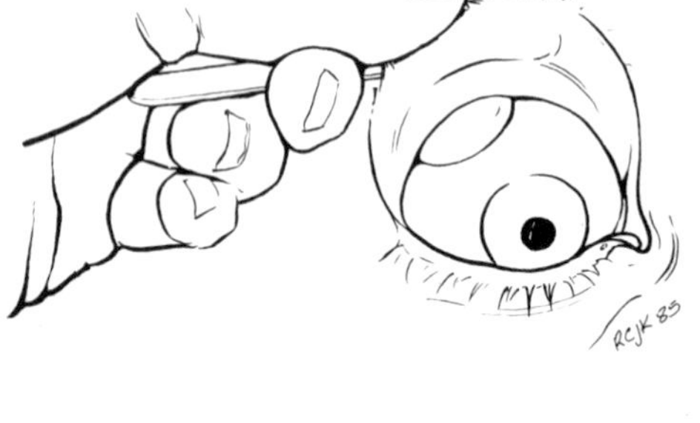

Fig. 5.3 Contact lens in the fornix revealed by single eversion.

4. Hold the lower lid down towards the lower orbital rim and inspect the lower cul-de-sac.

5. If the lens is not located, double eversion of the upper lid is needed (Figs 5.4a, b, c).

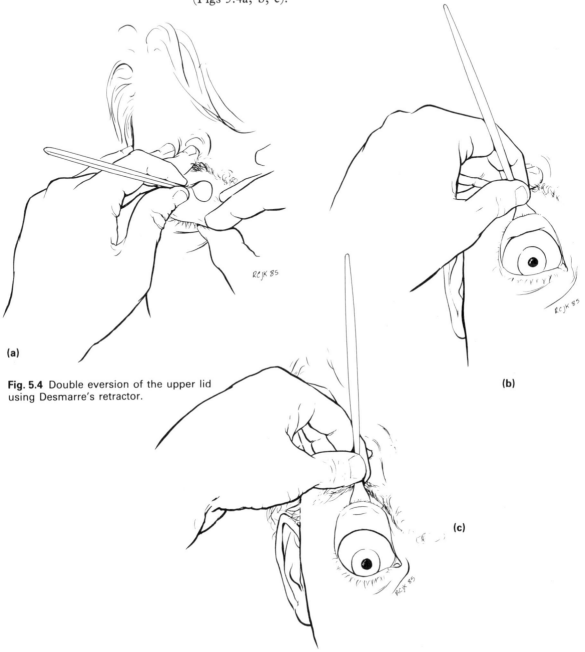

(a)

Fig. 5.4 Double eversion of the upper lid using Desmarre's retractor.

(b)

(c)

Treatment

1. When the lens has been located, place a cotton bud on the centre of the lens surface and slide it gently onto the cornea.

2. A suction cup can be used to remove the lens if necessary, or the patient may remove it as previously instructed by the fitter.

SUPERFICIAL BURNS

CHEMICAL BURNS

These should never be regarded as superficial.

Treatment
1. Immediate irrigation, to be continued for 15 minutes.
2. Apply antibiotic ointment.
3. See page 88.

THERMAL BURNS OF THE EYE
Treatment
1. Remove foreign material.
2. Irrigate gently.
3. Apply antibiotic ointment.
4. Apply sterile non-adhesive dressing.

THERMAL BURNS OF THE LIDS

Rapid lid closure and later swelling usually protects the eye in the acute phase.

Treatment
1. Apply a combined antibiotic ointment copiously over the burnt area.
2. Apply a sterile non-adhesive dressing.

ULTRAVIOLET BURNS

There is a latent period after exposure before symptoms arise, and there is severe photophobia. The patient may need topical anaesthetic drops for examination, and shows extensive punctate staining of the cornea with fluorescein.

Treatment
1. Apply a topical antibiotic and cycloplegic.
2. Avoid further topical anaesthetic.
3. Apply an eyepad.

CONJUNCTIVITIS

This is usually bilateral, because it is infectious and it is difficult to prevent contagion from one to the other eye. However, it is often asymmetrical. It can be bacterial, chlamydial or viral. There is a discharge; lids are stuck together in the morning. The visual acuity is unaffected except when discharge sweeps across the cornea.

If the conjunctivitis is unilateral, consider foreign body (FB) or sac obstruction. Diagnostic scraping and culture may be required.

Treatment
1. Moist swabbing to remove discharge.
2. Topical antibiotic drops (no steroid).
3. Avoid eye padding.
4. Refer if the condition has not settled in 1 week.

OPHTHALMIA NEONATORUM

This occurs within three weeks of birth. There is great danger of corneal involvement. It is commonly a chlamydial (TRIC), gonococcal, staphylococcal or pneumococcal infection. The lids are closed and may have pus under pressure behind them. Refer such cases urgently for in-patient care.

CONJUNCTIVAL OEDEMA (CHEMOSIS)

This is often allergic or caused by small flying insects in summer. It is persistent if constricted against the lid margin.

Treatment
1. Antibiotic drops.
2. Try to lift lids over to cover the swollen conjunctiva.
3. Support the closed lids with a pressure dressing.

BLEPHARITIS

The lids are sore and red. There is no conjunctival flush. It is associated with lash folliculitis, meibomitis. There is small risk of the infection spreading.

Blepharitis is recurrent, resistant and slow to respond. It needs weeks or months of therapy. There are often associated skin lesions, furunculosis, seborrhoea, eczema, impetigo, lid lice.

Treatment
1. Topical antibiotic ointment.
2. Culture for sensitivity if resistant.
3. Local heat.
4. Massage to express inspissated meibomian secretion.

STYE (HORDEOLUM)

This affects children more than adults. It is an infection of lash follicle or associated glands, commonly staphyloccocal. The symptoms are local pain and tenderness, and oedema of whole affected lid. The stye may point and discharge or may resolve.

Check urine for glucose.

Treatment
1. Topical antibiotic ointment.
2. May need systemic therapy if there is general toxicity.
3. Avoid surgery.

MEIBOMIAN CYSTS

These affect adults more than children. They may have an acute inflammatory onset, but usually this is slow enlargement of a hard lump a little apart from the lid margin.

Treat a meibomian cyst acutely as a stye.

ORBITAL ODEMA

In the absence of inflammatory signs, there is probably angioneurotic oedema.

Treatment is non-specific.

CONTACT DERMATITIS

This is due to sensitivity to a great variety of irritants. It is usually allergic, caused by pollens, cosmetics, local eye treatments. It can be induced by domestic and industrial fluids and gases, and is aggravated by rubbing and wetting by tears. The onset is fairly rapid. Symptoms are redness and scaling of lids.

Treatment
1. Remove the cause.
2. Apply local antihistamine and steroid.
3. If the patient is hypersensitive to all topical agents, he/she may need systemic treatment and sedatives.

EPISCLERITIS

Mild discomfort is experienced. There is a raised nodule on sclera with surrounding redness. Episcleritis is often recurrent.

Treatment
Topical steroids are usually effective.

SERIOUS CONDITIONS

Acute ocular inflammation
Acute iritis
Acute glaucoma
Herpes zoster ophthalmicus
Swelling and inflammation of periocular tissues and orbit

More extensive and deeper burns
All chemical burns
Blunt and perforating injuries
Orbital fractures
Rapid visual loss

ACUTE OCULAR INFLAMMATION

KERATITIS

The eye is closed, so testing visual acuity is difficult. When the eye is open, it is watery, so testing is still difficult. It sometimes needs topical anaesthetic to allow the patient to open the eye for reasonable examination.

If the epithelium is not intact, fluorescein will stain and may confirm diagnosis of abrasion, non-specific or herpetic (dendritic) ulcer.

Treatment

1. Apply antibiotic ointment and mydriatic (because of pain from pupil spasm).
2. Must avoid steroids if there is any possibility of herpetic cause.
3. Look for hypopyon, especially when the condition is suddenly worse a few days after onset.

EPIDEMIC KERATOCONJUNCTIVITIS (ADENOVIRUS)

The onset is acute. The disease is highly contagious. There is a danger of spread through first aid, A&E and ophthalmic units.

There is follicular conjunctivitis. The pre-auricular gland is enlarged and tender. The disease is self-limiting in several weeks and can leave corneal scarring. It is resistant to treatment.

Treatment

Oily tetracycline eye drops.

CORNEAL ULCER

More pain than conjunctivitis
Some photophobia
Vision affected if central
Gram-negative organisms are very dangerous. Look for greyish patch on cornea, and for a dull yellow stain with fluorescein.

Treatment

1. Topical antibiotic and cycloplegia.
2. Sub-conjunctival antibiotic if the condition is severe.
3. No topical steroid because the disease *may be due to the herpes simplex virus (dendritic ulcer)* which is potentiated by steroids.

HERPETIC ULCER

There is pain in excess of inflammation. The eye waters and exhibits photophobia. There is no corneal opacity at an early stage. The ulcer shows well when stained with fluorescein as a green branching (dendritic) pattern (Fig. 5.5).

Treatment
1. Topical acyclovir.
2. Cycloplegia.
3. NO STEROIDS.

CATARRHAL ULCER

This is commonly marginal, recurrent and often due to staphylococcal allergy. It is sometimes associated with aphthous buccal ulcers. It stains poorly with fluorescein.

Treatment
Topical antibiotic (and steroid drops, if the diagnosis is certain).

SCLERITIS

There is deep ocular pain. The subconjunctival area is dark red, diffuse and tender. There is usually a systemic collagenosis.

Treatment
1. Systemic steroids.
2. Other anti-inflammatory therapeutic agents.
3. Scleritis is not responsive to local therapy.

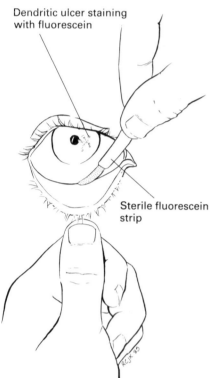

Dendritic ulcer staining with fluorescein

Sterile fluorescein strip

Fig. 5.5 Dendritic ulcer.

ACUTE IRITIS (Fig. 5.6)

The visual acuity is reduced: about 6/18, i.e. about halfway down the test chart. There is circumcorneal injection. Corneal surface reflection is unimpaired. There may be some corneal stromal oedema. There is aqueous flare. Iris details are concealed by aqueous flare and swelling of iris stroma.

The ciliary body is so close that it will usually be involved in the inflammation. So many cells are exuded from the ciliary capillaries that they are deposited in clumps on the back surface of the cornea, forming keratic precipitates (KP). They gravitate preferentially on the lower quadrant of the cornea, because this part of the cornea is directed upwards.

There is aching pain and tenderness of the globe. The iris swelling and spasm of the sphincter makes the pupil smaller. Adhesions form between the pupil and the surface of the lens (posterior synechiae). The iris is not usually in contact with the more peripheral lens, so adhesions are not formed except at the pupil.

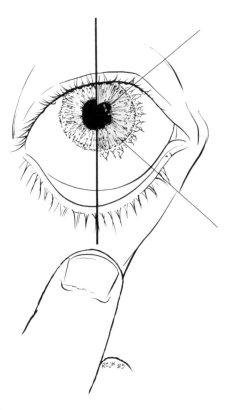

Fig. 5.6 Acute iritis.

Think of associated general conditions; especially spondylitis, gonorrhoea, Reiter's syndrome, AIDS.

Treatment
Atropine 1% and local steroid, but atropine has a prolonged effect so think of phenylephrine or homatropine as alternatives until diagnosis is confirmed.

These patients need to be investigated and treated in an ophthalmic unit. The presence of frank exudate in the anterior chamber (hypopyon) or vitreous (endophthalmitis) is an indication for urgent in-patient care.

ACUTE GLAUCOMA (Fig. 5.7)

Visual acuity is grossly affected; there may be no light perception. It is usually <6/60, i.e. no letters are read on the test chart. There is severe pain, which may cause vomiting and collapse. Absence of severe pain should not be taken to exclude the diagnosis.

Reflection from the corneal surface is steamy: this means oedema of the epithelium and this in turn means glaucoma until proved otherwise.

There is congestion of conjunctiva and circumcorneal vessels. The

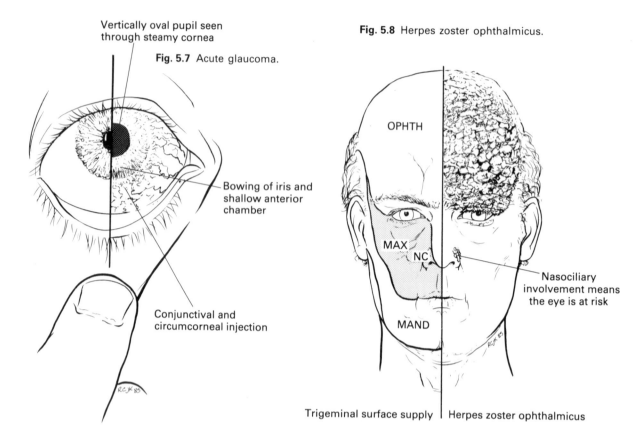

Vertically oval pupil seen through steamy cornea

Fig. 5.7 Acute glaucoma.

Fig. 5.8 Herpes zoster ophthalmicus.

Bowing of iris and shallow anterior chamber

Conjunctival and circumcorneal injection

OPHTH

MAX

NC

MAND

Nasociliary involvement means the eye is at risk

Trigeminal surface supply | Herpes zoster ophthalmicus

pupil is oval (vertically) and the anterior chamber is shallow. The disease is precipitated by darkness, distress, and death of a near relative. There are rainbow haloes around points of light.

Treatment

1. Miotics (pilocarpine 4%, eserine 0.5%) acetazolamide.
2. Peripheral iridectomy is needed if the condition is not quickly responsive.
3. The other eye may need prophylactic peripheral iridectomy.

HERPES ZOSTER OPHTHALMICUS (Fig. 5.8)

Severe pain without signs is experienced for 2–3 days. Then there is vesication and sub-epithelial infiltration. The pain and rash are strictly within the Vth nerve distribution. The disease is commoner in the old and frail. There is danger of keratitis if the nasociliary nerve is affected.

Look for vesicles on lower side of nose.

Treatment

1. Local toilet.
2. Topical antibiotic and steroid.

SWELLING AND INFLAMMATION OF PERIOCULAR TISSUES AND ORBIT

BLUNT TRAUMA

Oedema and haemorrhage cause exophthalmos and limitation of movement. The optic nerve can allow 5 mm of forward displacement without threat to function, but not more. If tissues are tense, decompression may be needed, but this requires ophthalmic consultation and a joint decision.

The levator aponeurosis can be torn by blunt trauma causing ptosis, especially in old people. Medial canthus disruption can cause lateral displacement of tissues.

Treatment
1. Sedative.
2. Avoid compression.
3. Residual deformity may require ophthalmic plastic surgery.

CAROTICOCAVERNOUS FISTULA (Fig. 5.9)

This may follow trauma, such as fracture of skull base. Onset is often sudden and spontaneous. Arterial blood under high pressure reverses

Fig. 5.9 Caroticocavernous fistula.

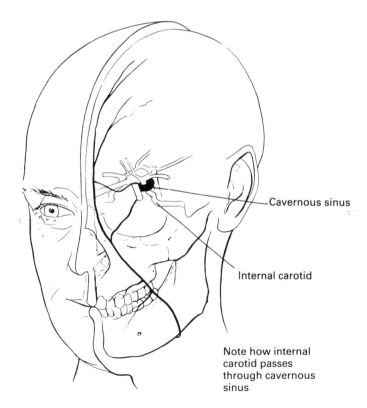

Cavernous sinus

Internal carotid

Note how internal carotid passes through cavernous sinus

the flow in the orbital veins, which are grossly engorged. The symptoms may present on the unaffected side or with bilateral signs:
– proptosis
– pulsation
– loud bruit over orbit

Treatment
Refer.

ACUTE DACRYOADENITIS

This is rare, and is usually part of a systemic disease. Pain is followed by tender swelling of the upper outer orbital tissues after a few hours. Redness and oedema may extent to the temple, resembling a lid abscess. The underlying conjunctiva is red and swollen. There is general malaise and fever. Think of mumps, glandular fever. The disease is unlikely to respond to antibiotics.

Treatment
Refer.

ACUTE DACRYOCYSTITIS (Fig. 5.10)

This can occur in neonates, in which case refer to the ophthalmologist. It occurs mostly in adults over middle age, predominating in females by 3:1. It may be acute or chronic: there may be a history of prolonged watery eye.

Fig. 5.10 Acute dacryocystitis.

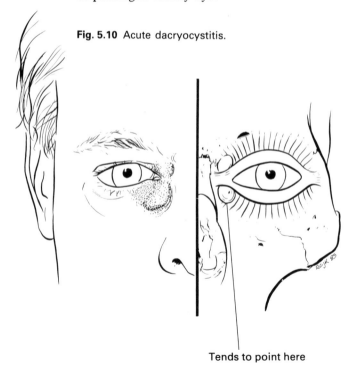

Tends to point here

The usual inflammatory signs appear and the onset is sudden. There is pain, tense swelling and redness at the medial canthus. Local cellulitis may perforate below the medial canthal ligament and may need drainage. There is oedema of the lower lid. The cause is often pneumococcal.

Treatment
1. Local heat.
2. Systemic and prophylactic topical antibiotics.
3. The patient may need planned ophthalmic surgery to relieve obstruction when quiescent (dacryocystogram, syringe and probe, dacryocystorhinostomy).

CAVERNOUS SINUS THROMBOSIS (Fig. 5.11)

There is rapid and dramatic spread of infection from orbital or facial sepsis. The onset is violent with trigeminal pain. There is pyrexia and severe malaise, proptosis, restricted movement (due to swelling and extraocular muscle palsies), congestion of conjunctiva and lids, and engorgement of retinal veins.

Fig. 5.11 Routes of infective spread in cavernous sinus thrombosis.

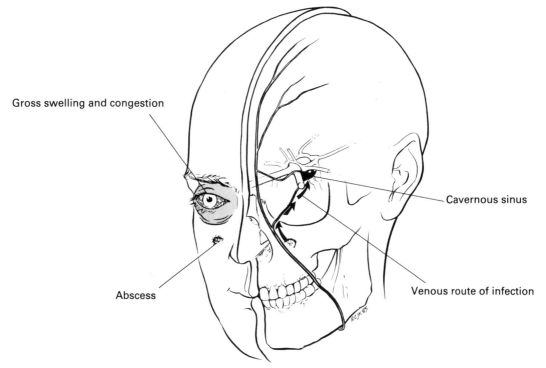

Gross swelling and congestion

Abscess

Cavernous sinus

Venous route of infection

Treatment
Intravenous antibiotics, and consider anticoagulants.

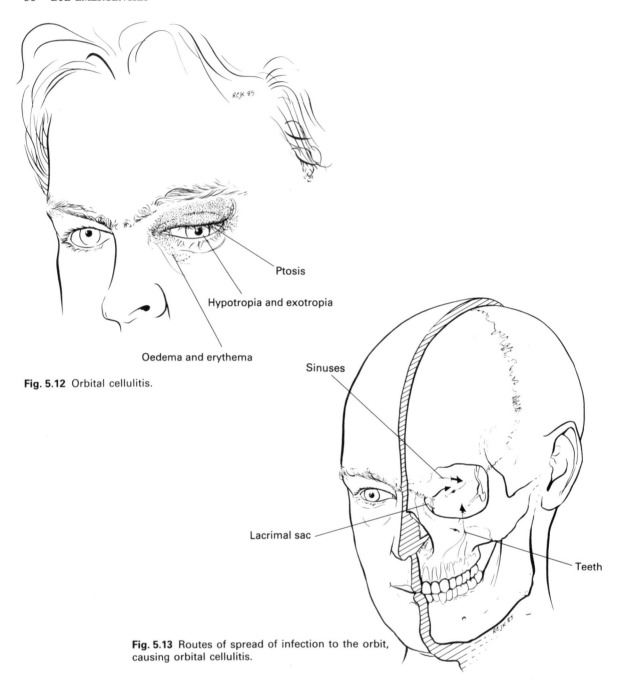

Fig. 5.12 Orbital cellulitis.

Ptosis

Hypotropia and exotropia

Oedema and erythema

Sinuses

Lacrimal sac

Teeth

Fig. 5.13 Routes of spread of infection to the orbit, causing orbital cellulitis.

ORBITAL CELLULITIS (Fig. 5.12)

This is always serious. There is spread of infection from an adjacent area (Fig. 5.13):
– sinuses
– teeth
– lacrimal sac or through the bloodstream. In children the infection usually spreads from the ethmoids.

Symptoms are:
- Pain, fever and toxicity
- Conjunctival congestion and oedema
- Brawny lid swelling
- Axial proptosis
- Restricted ocular movement
- Possible loss of vision

Treatment
1. Treat vigorously with systemic (i.e. intravenous) antibiotics.
2. ENT opinion and treatment.
3. Protect the cornea from exposure.
4. Apply topical antibiotic ointment.
5. Consider possible optic nerve compression.
6. May need drainage to decompress.

ORBITAL TRAUMA

When there is a penetrating wound:
- be sure there is no CSF fistula
- think of foreign body.
Wood fragments are often surprisingly large from pencils, branches and arrows, but do not show well on X-ray (see Figure 4.32a).

Treatment
1. Remove foreign body if it is:
- vegetable matter
- anterior, or
- has ragged sharp edges.
2. Leave foreign body if it is:
- inert
- posterior
- smooth.
3. Culture wound and foreign body.
4. Suspect a fracture and refer as appropriate. (See also pages 93, 106.)

EXTENSIVE AND DEEP BURNS

THERMAL BURNS

The eye may closed at first, but contraction of scar tissue can endanger the eye by exposure.

It is difficult in burns of the face and lids to determine whether the burn involves the full thickness of the skin. Early tarsorraphy may be required and a skin graft over the whole burned area, covering the eye.

Treatment
1. Apply a combined antibiotic ointment copiously over the burnt area, covering the eye.
2. Refer to an ophthalmic unit if the injury is localised or a burns unit if extensive.

CHEMICAL BURNS

These should never be regarded as superficial. They require immediate irrigation from the nearest water source. All staff need to be informed of the urgency of these cases so that they are treated without delay.

The lids have to be held forcibly apart. Irrigation needs to be continued for 15 minutes.

Burns usually mainly affect the lower fornix. Lime particles get under the upper lid too.

Treatment
1. Instil topical anaesthetic.
2. Apply a facial nerve block if lid spasm prevents view. (Absence of pain does not mean the burn is mild; the eye may be anaesthetic as a result of the burn.)
3. Remove particles with swab or blunt forceps.
4. Irrigate freely again for 20 minutes with fluid from intravenous drip bottles. Litmus paper may monitor the efficiency of irrigation.
5. Instil antibacterial eye drops as a prophylactic; instil mydriatic/cycloplegic to prevent pupil spasm; topical ascorbic or citric acid may be helpful.
6. Acetazolamide tablets to reduce intraocular pressure in severe anterior segment burns.
7. Test and record vision.
8. Apply a sterile pad
9. Refer urgently to ophthalmologist.

BLUNT AND PERFORATING INJURIES

BLUNT INJURY

Blunt trauma can cause rupture of the globe or tears of its internal structures. The damage may be revealed by obvious intraocular haemorrhage, tears of the iris, cataract or dislocation of the lens. Damage to the posterior segment of the eye may be less evident. A clear view may be prevented by diffuse bleeding in the anterior chamber or vitreous, but tears of the retina or choroid, or detachment of the retina, are common.

Haemorrhage from the choroid can spread in the suprachoroidal space.

Multiple areas of damage are likely, and these are usually anatomically related, so an appropriate search must be made during the examination to establish the extent.

A rupture of the sclera is easily concealed by sub-conjunctival bleeding and must be considered in any severe blunt injury, particularly in older patients.

Tears of the iris (Fig. 5.14) either involve the pupil, when they cut through the sphincter and extend in a radial direction, or the root,

Fig. 5.14 Tears of the iris.

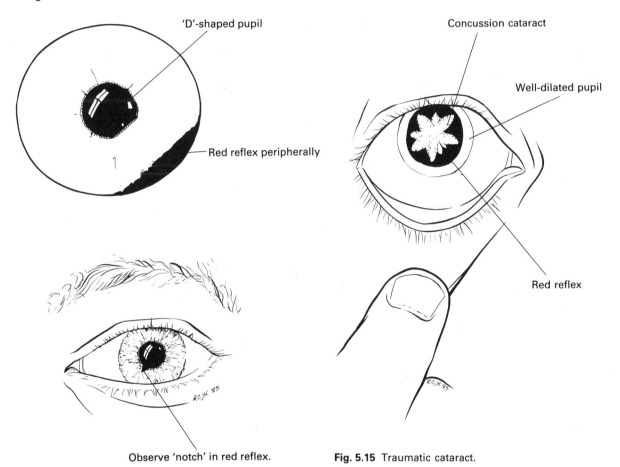

'D'-shaped pupil

Red reflex peripherally

Concussion cataract

Well-dilated pupil

Red reflex

Observe 'notch' in red reflex.

Fig. 5.15 Traumatic cataract.

when they disinsert the periphery, causing the pupil to be D-shaped and often permitting a red reflex to be seen through the periphery.

Cataract (Fig. 5.15) often shows as a lace or petal pattern in the centre of the posterior cortex of the lens. At first it is clearly defined, but later becomes an amorphous disc. A dislocated lens (Fig. 5.16) can no longer support the iris, which is tremulous on any movement of the eye. This is a sure sign of displacement of the lens. A more complete dislocation can reveal the equatorial edge of the lens in the pupil, part of the fundus can be seen through the phakic and part through the aphakic area.

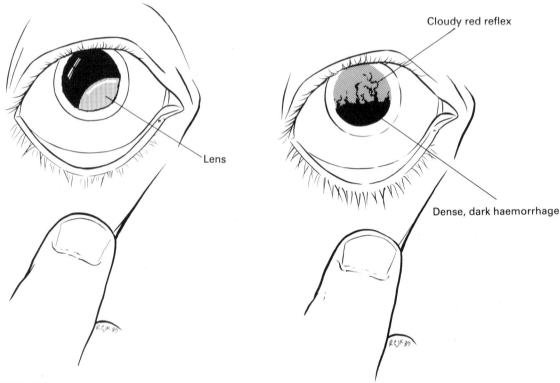

Fig. 5.16 Dislocated lens.

Fig. 5.17 Vitreous haemorrhage, as seen with an ophthalmoscope.

Complete vitreous haemorrhage abolishes the red reflex and appears almost black immediately behind a clear lens. When less complete, it often gravitates below with fronds extending upwards from the main mass. Fundus details are hazy even in places where there is still some red reflex.

Traumatic tears of the retina (Fig. 5.17) are seen near its periphery at the site of injury or directly opposite. They may be too peripheral to be seen with the direct ophthalmoscope even when the clinician is deliberately looking as obliquely as possible through the dilated pupil. In the presence of haemorrhage there is a risk of retinal detachment as organisation commences. Choroidal tears (Fig. 5.18) are typically crescent-shaped and sited a little away from, but concentric with, the optic disc. Immediately after injury they may be concealed by haemorrhage.

Management
All severe blunt injuries and those less severe but with intraocular haemorrhage should be referred.

Pale crescent surrounded by blood

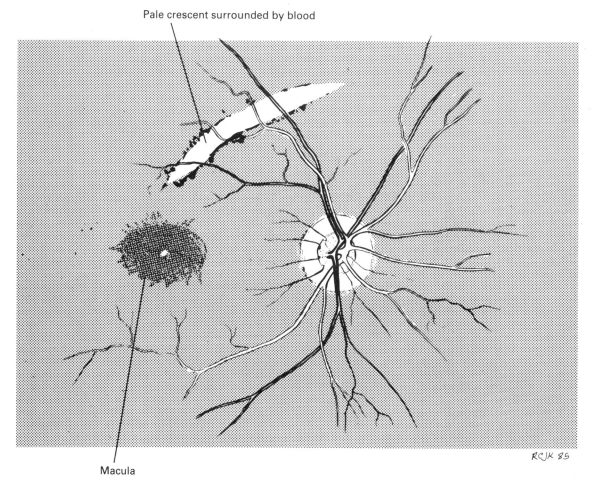

Macula

RCJK 85

Fig. 5.18 Choroidal tear.

PERFORATING INJURY

A gross perforation of the globe with loss of ocular contents should be suspected if the lids of the injured eye appear sunken or if there is blood clot between the lid margins. Great care is needed in any attempt to open the lids to avoid increasing the damage.

A leaking corneal wound is associated with a shallow or absent anterior chamber, pupil displacement or iris prolapse. Iris outside the eye may have lost its pigment and mislead the examiner to think it is a fibrin clot. Wounds at or across the corneal margin (limbus) are likely to be sealed by uveal tissue or blood. Scleral perforations are usually concealed by blood, but the black uveal pigment may be visible enough to make the diagnosis possible.

Deeper penetrations of the cornea will involve the lens. Cataract is obvious very soon, as aqueous is absorbed into the lens fibres causing them to swell and opacify. Sometimes the pupil contracts to cover an area of lens damage, and in all cases of perforating injury it is necessary to exclude this possibility by careful examination, dilating the pupil with a mydriatic when required.

Management

All perforating injuries, however small, need to be referred.

Suspect the presence of an intraocular foreign body if:
– a hammer and chisel were being used
– there was any breakage of metal
– there was any broken glass

Open perforating wounds and intraocular foreign bodies need urgent referral.

Immediate treatment

1. Pad the eye without disturbance.
2. Give a broad-spectrum antibiotic.
3. Tetanus prophylaxis.

Scleral perforations and ruptures may be concealed by sub-conjunctival blood. They are managed in a similar way.

Lacerations of the orbit may be accompanied by orbital haemorrhage and raised intraorbital pressure. This may threaten the ophthalmic circulation, and urgent decompression may be required. Acetazolamide given intravenously may be a useful emergency measure.

OPTIC NERVE DAMAGE

Falling on to a pointed object may cause direct damage to the optic nerve, but frequently the damage is due to forward movement of the optic nerve in its canal, which disrupts the small blood vessels supplying the nerve, causing ischaemic optic atrophy (Fig. 5.19). This

Fig. 5.19 Scheme showing the blood supply to the optic nerve (right side, viewed laterally).

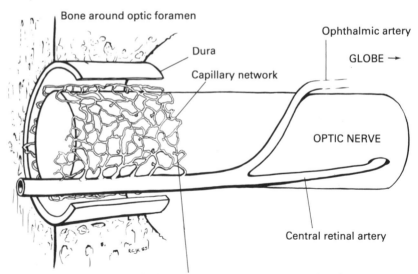

These weak vessels are liable to tear when there is relative shearing movement between the nerve and its surrounding tissues.

causes immediate blindness in the affected eye, but only showing pallor of the optic disc after some weeks. The penetrating object may indeed pass through the orbit and into the cranial cavity, making a full ophthalmic and neurological assessment as well as an X-ray essential to exclude retention of a foreign body or penetration of the roof.

Organic foreign bodies can induce severe and persistent cellulitis.

Be sure that you always recheck the pupil reactions and visual acuity when there is a possibility of such damage. Refer for further assessment.

ORBITAL FRACTURE

Suspect a fracture in orbital injury with:
– bruising
– emphysema of the
  lid tissues
– infraorbital
  anaesthesia
– double vision

In the early period after orbital injury, swelling may conceal the presence of a fracture of either the margin or orbital wall.

Haematoma will restrict movement, and it is very difficult to determine if there is going to prove to be muscle incarceration in a 'blow-out' fracture line.

It has been the fashion to repair such cases early, but more conservative management has shown that function in most cases is recovered spontaneously.

The casualty officer should be aware of the possibilities and alert the ophthalmic and maxillofacial units at an early stage so that the correct management can be planned.

If fracture is diagnosed:

1. Advise the patient not to blow the nose forcibly, because of the risk of causing surgical emphysema.

2. Refer for admission any patient with restricted eye movements.

3. Extensive disruption of the orbit leaves a very poor cosmetic appearance, if not properly treated.

4. Urgent decompression may be required.

The orbit is limited anteriorly by the orbital septum and elsewhere by the orbital walls. Oedema and haemorrhage may cause such an increase in pressure as to endanger the blood supply to the eye.

Decompression is obtained by incision through the orbital septum below the brow and through the lower lid (Fig. 5.20).

Surgical emphysema occurs in fracture of the ethmoid (lamina papyracea).

Loss of sensation in the inferior orbital nerve distribution is found in fracture of the orbital floor.

The naso-lacrimal duct is obstructed in fractures of the nose or medial orbit.

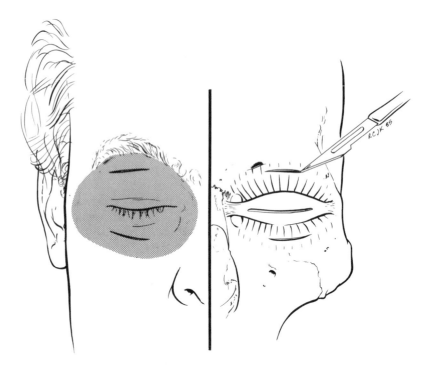

Fig. 5.20 Incisions for decompression of the orbit.

Oedema and haematoma may:
- obscure bony displacement
- conceal displacement of the eye.

Plain and tomographic X-rays can show orbital fractures. Computerised tomography (CT scan) can show both bony and soft tissue damage. These are especially well seen on coronal tomographic scans.

Many fractures do not restrict eye movement or cause significant disfigurement, so they do not demand surgical intervention.

RAPID VISUAL LOSS

VITREOUS HAEMORRHAGE

This may occur spontaneously, as well as after trauma. Proliferative diabetic retinopathy may present with vitreous haemorrhage as the first cause of visual disturbance. Other retinal vascular conditions may also present in this way. Always think of retinal breaks as a possible cause, which may lead on to retinal detachment.

Management
Close observation of all cases is required until the cause has been established. These patients need proper ophthalmic assessment.

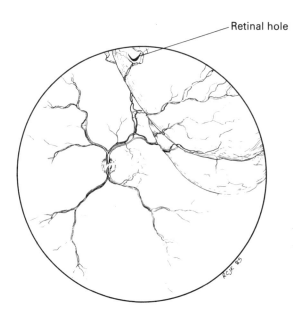

Retinal hole

Fig. 5.21 Retinal detachment.

RETINAL DETACHMENT

(Fig. 5.21) There is usually a recent history of floaters, flashes of light and a curtain across the vision. Retinal detachment is recognised by ophthalmoscopic examination with a dilated pupil. The retina is grey, and the retinal hole or break is seen as red. It will show on ultrasonography or computerised tomography (CT scan) if the fundus cannot be seen.

Treatment
Specialised ophthalmic surgical management is required to:
1. Seal retinal breaks (by cryopexy or photocoagulation).
2. Prevent continued vitreous traction (by indentation, encirclement or intravitreal surgery).
3. Referral is most urgent when macular function is threatened.

DISCIFORM MACULAR DEGENERATION

(Fig. 5.22) This may present with a sudden severe impairment or complete loss of central vision of one eye, but retention of the peripheral field. It may be difficult to see without dilating the pupil and, even then, this may only show macular oedema with an area a little larger than the optic disc. Usually there is some surrounding haemorrhage and this may predominate. The patient needs further ophthalmic examination.

When one eye has been affected by this condition, there is a probability that the other eye will be similarly affected within 10 years. Patients who have sustained a disciform degeneration in one eye and subsequently experience central visual disturbance in the other should be considered as an emergency, because some are amenable to laser treatment in the prodromal phase.

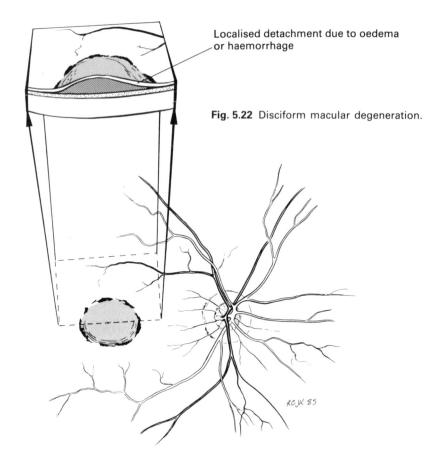

Localised detachment due to oedema or haemorrhage

Fig. 5.22 Disciform macular degeneration.

CENTRAL RETINAL ARTERIAL THROMBOSIS

Sudden painless loss of vision is experienced. Retinal arteries are very narrow, collapse on slight pressure and may show 'shunting'. The macula shows as a cherry-red spot against the white background of infarcted retina. Associated conditions are:
- hypertension
- atheroma
- heart disease
- arteritis

There is no return of function if the retinal artery is obstructed for more than six hours. Optic disc atrophy shows after several weeks. Branch occlusion is always embolic and is more likely to resolve.

Treatment
1. Intravenous acetazolamide.
2. Massage of the globe.
3. Anticoagulants can be tried.
4. Intravenous steroids if arteritis. (Check ESR).
5. Long-term aspirin.

OPTIC NERVE ISCHAEMIA (GIANT CELL ARTERITIS)

Headache (temporal, occipital) is experienced. There is tenderness over affected arteries. Euphoria is common. ESR is mostly raised, but the disease may present without these associated features.

Clinical findings
1. Defective afferent pupil response.
2. Small vessels of optic nerve are affected.
3. Slight yellowish pallor of disc.
4. Central retinal artery and fundus are normal.

Treatment
1. Intravenous steroids.
2. High-dose steroids till ESR returns to normal.
3. Continued for months and monitored.

METHYL ALCOHOL POISONING

There is sudden bilateral loss of vision, inactive dilated pupils, swelling of optic discs, localised retinal oedema and engorgement of veins, acidosis and dehydration.

Treatment
1. Correct acidosis and dehydration.
2. Then give diuretic.
3. Then give ethyl alcohol.

HYSTERICAL BLINDNESS

The patient exhibits an indifferent attitude. The history is vague and labile. The patient claims no light perception but avoids visible hazards.

The pupil reactions are normal, but remember that true cortical blindness also shows normal pupil reactions. There is retained opto-kinetic nystagmus. Cortical visual evoked responses should be normal.

Treatment
Confirm diagnosis in consultation with ophthalmologist or neurologist and refer for psychiatric management.

6

Further management

In this chapter further management of more severe ophthalmic conditions will be described. Traumatic conditions are considered first.

Blunt injury
Perforating injury
Intraocular foreign bodies
Sympathetic ophthalmitis
Burns
Orbital fractures
Retinal detachment
Acute glaucoma
Chronic glaucoma
Proliferative diabetic retinopathy
Vitreous haemorrhage
Disciform macular degeneration
Central retinal arterial obstruction
Central retinal vein obstruction

BLUNT INJURY

HYPHAEMA

The patient is usually admitted for bed rest and observation. A careful examination will be made for other contusion damage which may require early or later treatment. The source of bleeding is commonly from the iris root or anterior face of the ciliary body, and in severe injuries there is a significant risk of secondary haemorrhage. This serious complication is more likely in an eye which remains flushed and irritable at the third day after injury, but the risk may be reduced by topical steroids.

Should secondary bleeding occur, the anterior chamber rapidly fills with blood and there is a sharp rise of intraocular pressure. This may respond to oral acetazolamide (Diamox), but if unrelieved the increased pressure causes loss of vision by restricting the intraocular circulation. In such cases a peripheral iridectomy may be needed to overcome pupillary obstruction, bring down the pressure and permit the blood to be absorbed more quickly.

Speed in controlling the pressure is needed not only to prevent blindness from circulatory obstruction, but also to prevent damage to the corneal endothelium and bloodstaining of the corneal stroma.

TEARS OR DIALYSIS OF THE IRIS

These will not be repaired unless they are the cause of symptoms of light scatter or diplopia, or in the course of anterior segment surgery such as the removal of a concussion cataract.

DISLOCATION OF THE LENS

This may cause intolerable interference with vision, and late complications of iritis or glaucoma. The lens can remain clear, but its removal may be as justifiable as for cataract. If the lens is much displaced, it may be necessary to fixate it by a needle before proceding to remove it.

CONCUSSION CATARACT

This too may cause sufficient visual disturbance to justify its extraction. It can be removed using either the intracapsular or extracapsular method, with precautions to avoid vitreous complications. The procedure can be very similar to the removal of a senile cataract by either method. The insertion of an intraocular lens is indicated, provided it can be properly secured, because this gives the best prospect of regaining binocular stereoscopic vision.

Intracapsular extraction may need no modification, provided the anterior chamber is free of vitreous, but the surgeon must be sure of this and avoid any possibility of incarceration of tissue into the wound by performing an anterior vitrectomy, if necessary. Incarceration leads to traction on intraocular structures, an irritable eye and a high risk of retinal detachment.

The standard extracapsular method cannot be applied when the lens is dislocated. The dislocated lens and damaged vitreous can be removed posteriorly through the pars plana 4 mm behind the corneal margin using an infusion and suction cutter. A suitable intraocular lens may be implanted through a corneal incision after this is completed.

Provided that the retina has not been injured by the contusion, there is a good prognosis for the recovery of vision.

VITREOUS HAEMORRHAGE AFTER CONTUSION

This implies internal damage affecting the retina, with a high risk of retinal detachment as the blood organises and contraction develops. In blunt trauma the retinal break is usually at the vitreous base due to the distortion of the globe at the site of injury.

The treatment of haemorrhage and retinal detachment will be discussed below.

PERFORATING EYE INJURIES

Early repair must be performed in almost all cases. All parts of the eye are accessible to primary microsurgical repair. The closure of corneoscleral wounds is made accurate and watertight. This reduces or prevents many complications such as infection, vascularisation and downgrowth of epithelium through the wound, which then spreads widely within the eye. Closure must be watertight, because a persistently shallow anterior chamber encourages progressive closure of the drainage angle, leading to intractable glaucoma.

Closing of the wound is only part of the primary microsurgery. In addition, the iris can be repaired, a traumatic cataract removed, haemorrhage cleared away, and vitreous and retinal problems prevented or repaired.

Iris repair can result in a functioning iris diaphragm and a central round pupil. This is more than a cosmetic advantage: it has optical advantages, and a complete diaphragm helps to establish an anterior chamber of normal depth, preventing adhesion to the corneal wound and obstruction of the drainage angle. 10/0 polypropylene is the most suitable material for use at present, because it is almost inert and very long-lasting.

TRAUMATIC CATARACT

Traumatic cataract after perforation of the lens capsule is characterised by flocculent swelling of the lens cortex, and this adds to the possibility of adhesions and angle obstruction; uveitis ensues, with threat of a stormy convalesence. It is expedient to remove as much of the lens cortex as possible at the time of primary repair using simple aspiration or a suction cutter. The suction cutter can, at the same time, remove clotted blood and any vitreous prolapse. This may result in a much quieter clinical course and early return of function. Binocular vision can often be regained by wearing a contact lens on the injured eye or by secondary implantation of an intraocular lens.

INTRAOCULAR FOREIGN BODIES

Depending on the nature of the injury, foreign materials may be retained within the eye. Some will be noxious to intraocular tissues and they may also carry infection into the eye. Their presence should always be suspected in penetrating injury and steps taken to confirm or exclude them.

Deep corneal foreign bodies need careful removal at the slit-lamp, but, if there is any possibility that they have penetrated the full thickness, the patient must be taken to the operating theatre and the foreign body removed under the operating microscope. There is a great danger that an intact lens will be damaged if the anterior chamber is lost in the course of removal. Such a complication can alter the prognosis from a quick and full recovery if the lens remains undamaged to a disastrous series of events from which the patient may not regain binocular vision and, at worst, could lose that eye and become blind in the second eye from sympathetic ophthalmitis.

Foreign bodies which have penetrated further into the eye may be visible on examination, particularly when the slit-lamp is used. Others may be demonstrated and localised by X-rays, CT scan, electro-acoustic detectors and ultrasonography. Accurate localisation is essential in planning removal of the foreign bodies with the least surgical trauma.

Organic materials are very difficult to demonstrate and localise for removal. A persistently irritable eye after perforation often proves to contain dirty organic matter.

Glass and some metal fragments are sufficiently inert that it may be safer to leave them in situ rather than expose the eye to greater risk in attempting their removal.

Ferrous and copper-containing foreign bodies almost always lead to metallosis; siderosis in the case of iron and chalcosis from copper. Both are destructive to the function of the eye over a period of time. Accurate localisation of these foreign bodies is essential and then their safe removal can be planned.

The magnetic properties of some foreign bodies may be used in their removal: this method applies particularly to those situated anterior to the equator of the eye. Special pulsed magnets are available. Intraoperative electroacoustic localisation is helpful in confirming the exact position of the foreign body and permits the site of incision to be planned for its atraumatic removal.

Now that fine intravitreal instruments are available, more and more foreign bodies, whether magnetic or not, are amenable to removal under direct vision. Those in the anterior segment may be approached and removed through a limbal incision, but any placed posterior to the iris diaphragm may best be approached through the pars plana. Intravitreal 20 gauge instruments can provide illumination, infusion, suction, cutting and dissection, as well as a wide choice of forceps designed for grasping different types and sizes of foreign body.

Small fragments can be removed through the pars plana, but some are too large for the 20 gauge opening. As most of these will have caused disruption of the lens on entry, traumatic cataract and vitreous haemorrhage will need to be cleared by suction cutting before the foreign body is exposed and grasped. Rather than attempting to take them through the pars plana (even if the incision is enlarged) and risk losing them at that point, they can be manipulated through the pupil into the anterior chamber and more safely removed under direct vision through a limbal incision.

SYMPATHETIC OPHTHALMITIS

This devastating condition is much less common since repair became more accurate by using the operating microscope, and since steroid therapy enabled the inflammatory complications of perforating injury to be controlled.

The condition is a chronic granulomatous panuveitis which, although there are rare exceptions, occurs after penetrating injuries have damaged the uveal tissues, causing pigment granules to become extracellular and excite an immune response. This can lead on to the inflammatory destruction of the entire uveal tissue in the injured eye and, after a short 'incubation period', to a similar destruction of the uveal tissue of the uninjured eye, rendering them both blind. The condition is even worse than that, because the patient may also suffer deafness from coincident cochlear damage.

It must always be looked upon as a very serious disease, but when recognised early and treated immediately and vigorously the prognosis is greatly improved. It is essential to maintain adequate dilatation of the pupils and to control the inflammation with intensive steroid therapy. Betamethasone eyedrops are instilled four-hourly, with simultaneous large doses of systemic steroid. Treatment must be continued at a full maintenance level for at least six months after the last evidence of active uveitis.

BURNS

Thermal burns
Chemical burns
Extensive burns involving face and eyelids

INTRODUCTION

A description has already been given of the treatment of minor burns in the A&E department. The urgency of treatment needs further emphasis in the management of chemical burns, which may cause progressive damage from the continued presence of the chemical agent. This possibility needs to be determined at the outset and, where necessary, irrigation is continued and foreign debris removed for as long as there is any possibility of continued chemical action.

In all cases the next requirement is examination of the eye and its surroundings to determine the degree of damage and plan the management.

There are immediate and late problems to be considered, and it is helpful to consider separately the damage to the eye and the damage to the surrounding tissues. Each of these has different implications: the eye may suffer directly from the injury or later from lack of protection from the lids. If, as is often the case, the eye has been protected by reflex closure of the lids, much effort will be necessary to keep the eye protected from mechanical damage, dryness and infection.

THERMAL BURNS OF THE EYE

These can produce damage ranging from minor epithelial oedema to necrosis of tissue, depending on the heat source, the duration of exposure and the area of contact. It is possible for the moisture on the surface of the eye to protect it momentarily from a splash of molten metal, allowing the liquid to drop into the lower fornix where it is retained, solidifies and causes severe destruction. If the cornea is affected, it is almost always in its lower half.

The line of demarcation between necrotic and viable tissue is usually clearly shown by the limit of vascular engorgement. The extent of limbal damage is noted. If there is associated displacement of the pupil, then secondary glaucoma is very likely.

The more frequent problems of thermal burns of the eye are loss of vision due to scarring on the visual axis or irregular astigmatism when more peripheral scars contract.

BURNS OF THE LID MARGIN

The sudden reflex closure of the lids and elevation of the globe may protect the eye but cause the damage to be more severe at the lid margin. This may not affect the motility of the lids, and after healing the eye may appear to be well protected from exposure. These burns can, however, cause much permanent discomfort and watering by thinning of the lid structure, disturbance of the mucocutaneous junction, destruction of the meibomian ducts and damage to the lash follicles. The absence of the normal lid structure causes the tears to overflow. Aberrant lashes scratch the surface of the eye and compound the long-term problem. At the inner canthus the lacrimal puncta and canaliculi may be destroyed, causing intractable epiphora.

Plastic surgery to reconstruct the lids is difficult in these scarred conditions and is usually planned after the full extent of the problem is established.

CHEMICAL BURNS OF THE EYE

As already stated, the severity of chemical burns is variable according to the nature of the chemical, its concentration and penetrating capacity, the duration of contact and its reaction with the tissue components. Gases are less injurious than liquids or solid particles.

In general, acids coagulate the surface tissues, becoming neutralised and creating their own barrier to further penetration.

Sulphuric acid is particularly damaging because of its dehydrating effect.

Hydrofluoric acid and many alkalis penetrate deeply and have a prolonged effect, being held in the tissues to be released slowly and cause continuing damage.

Examination at hospital

Provided that in chemical burns irrigation and debridement have been efficiently carried out, the first consideration is a careful examination to establish the damage and plan the treatment. After the history has been taken and the visual acuity checked, the examination in cases of both chemical and thermal burns is similar.

Intense pain and blepharospasm often persist, making examination and treatment very difficult. (Sulphur dioxide, ammonia compounds and to a lesser extent other alkalis can cause anaesthesia, but this is associated with a worse prognosis.)

The structures which require particular consideration are the cornea, all parts of the conjunctiva and the lid margins. The cornea must be examined to establish the degree, area and depth of damage. Slit-lamp biomicroscopy with the use of sterile fluorescein or bengal rose will show the amount of epithelial damage.

Stromal damage can also be judged on the slit-lamp and by testing the corneal sensitivity. Pitting or faceting of the surface in thermal burns must imply deep, probably full-thickness damage. Full-thickness oedema of the stroma in chemical burns will almost always indicate deeper diffusion and intraocular involvement.

The conjunctiva should also be examined using vital staining. Any foreign debris should be removed on sight. Progressive degrees of damage are shown by hyperaemia, oedema, ischaemia, coagulation and necrosis.

The examination of the lid margins should take into account all its features, the mucocutaneous junction, the meibomian ducts, the lashes and the lacrimal ducts.

If the patient is unable to tolerate a proper examination, local or general anaesthesia is used. An operation consent form is completed with permission for any necessary surgery to be undertaken.

Classification

After the examination has been completed, the severity of the burn is classified (Table 6.1) so that management can be planned and the prognosis established. The condition of the cornea and conjunctiva are most important in the assessment of ultimate ocular function and they are best considered separately.

Table 6.1 Classification of burn severity

Grade	Cornea	Conjunctiva	Prognosis
I	Epithelial damage	No ischaemia	Good
II	Hazy, but iris details still seen	Ischaemia less than half at limbus	Good
III	Total epithelial loss Stromal haze Iris details obscured	Ischaemia affects $\frac{1}{3}$ to $\frac{1}{2}$ at limbus	Doubtful Vision reduced Perforation rare
IV	Opaque No view of iris or pupil	Ischaemia affects more than $\frac{1}{2}$ at limbus	Poor Prolonged treatment

Treatment

The aim is to secure and maintain comfortable vision. The patient is made as comfortable as possible with appropriate sedation. The cornea needs to be protected against further damage. Measures are taken to prevent or control infection. Cultures are taken frequently to detect and identify any pathogenic organisms. Steps are taken to prevent adhesions forming between two contiguous burned surfaces.

It is useful to consider the management of non-progressive and progressive burns separately.

Treatment of non-progressive thermal and chemical burns

In most cases treatment can be confined to the use of a topical antibiotic ointment. Steroids must be used with discretion; they can be very useful in reducing an excessive vascular response, but can lead to rapid softening of damaged corneal stroma in the presence of limbal ischaemia. The Walser shell is helpful in preventing adhesions.

Necrotic tissue should be removed; if the area is small, it can be left uncovered, but larger areas should be covered by a conjunctival flap from the upper fornix of the same eye or a free conjunctival graft from the other. Mucosal grafts are better reserved for the later stages of treatment except in desperate cases.

Emergency corneal grafting (keratoplasty) can be effective if there is an area of localised corneal necrosis and may prevent corneal vascularisation. Usually keratoplasty and plastic surgery to the lids and conjunctiva are performed as planned procedures after all inflammation has subsided.

Apart from the complicated and slow recovery of eyes with extensive limbal damage, glaucoma must be anticipated and treatment adjusted accordingly.

Treatment of progressive burns

Alkali burns are frequent, and many are clinically progressive. The prognostic classification is essential in determining management. In some Grade II and all more serious burns treatment must be directed to the removal of any residual noxious agent even if this means removal of the tissue containing it. In these severe burns local steroids must not be used, because of the risk of rapid softening and corneal perforation.

All cases need topical antibiotic and mydriasis. Glaucoma is frequent and needs special monitoring. Acetazolamide may be useful prophylactically. In some cases the sub-conjunctival injection of the patient's own blood may serve as a readily available, sterile, buffered fluid compatible with the tissues and serving to separate tissues, dilute and neutralise residual chemical and prevent its further spread.

Treatment of extensive burns involving face and eyelids

Neglected burns around the eye can result in serious deformity and blindness from the complications of exposure.

Antimicrobial control is all-important, and repeated cultures are necessary from the skin and conjunctival sac so that prompt and effective antibiotic treatment can be given. Burns are at first free from bacteria, those present having been killed by the heat or chemical, but soon the dead tissue and exudate become heavily colonised unless effective measures are taken to prevent this. The organisms are present before there is clinical evidence of infection. The application of a cream of mafenide acetate or 0.5% silver nitrate and 0.2% chlorhexidine is advocated as an antiseptic dressing. Laboratory controls of electrolyte balance are required for extensive burns.

At first, oedema of the lids protects the eyes, but as this subsides the eyelids may retract and expose the cornea. Local treatment, with antibiotic ointment and artificial tears, must be frequent and attentive. Bandage contact lenses or a shaped scleral ring may help in some cases. The cornea must be examined carefully for exposure changes, and treatment must be augmented vigorously if any ulceration is seen or frank infection occurs.

Protective skin grafting may be required and, because of the tendency for contraction of tissues to draw the lids apart, the graft may cover them completely for reopening when healing is complete.

ORBITAL FRACTURES

Most patients show a rapid recovery of ocular movement during the first few days after injury, so immediate surgery is not indicated.

Surgery is indicated if:
- double vision persists for 5 days when the patient is looking ahead or in down gaze
- enophthalmos exceeds 2 mm
- there is obvious fixation of the globe
- there is a large prolapse into the antrum shown on X-ray

The surgical repair is in the province of the maxillofacial surgeon and is usually delayed for a few days to allow oedema to subside.

BLOW-OUT FRACTURE OF THE ORBITAL FLOOR

The orbital floor is repaired by securing an implant over the defect after incising through the lower lid at the level of the floor and dissecting between the orbital periosteum and the orbital floor. The periosteum is elevated and gentle traction is exerted to ease the prolapsed tissues back into the orbit. The implant may be of autogenous bone, but more usually is made from soft silicone rubber.

Extensive disruption of the orbital floor may require access from within the antrum by using a Caldwell-Luc approach. Packing of the cavity is avoided, if possible.

If there is muscle entrapment:
- wait for oedema to subside
- lower orbital rim is approached through an incision several millimetres below the lid margin, through skin and muscle
- periosteum is elevated and trapped tissues are released
- the gap is covered by a small implant of silicon, polyamide or gelatin film
- larger implants risk damage to the optic nerve and extrusion
  For larger defects:
- approach from antrum as well as the orbit
- use a modified Caldwell-Luc procedure
- retain the anterior wall of the antrum to use in repair of the orbital floor

---

NASO-ORBITAL FRACTURES

When these are severe, they may involve the naso-lacrimal duct, causing a persistent dacrocystitis.

MORE COMPOUND INJURIES

These can involve extensive damage to the cranial base, the paranasal sinuses and the jaws. They require a multidisciplinary approach with neurosurgical, maxillofacial, plastic and ophthalmic teams contributing to the restoration of function and satisfactory appearance. This combined approach reduces the time in hospital and late complications. This primary approach can prevent the need for further surgical procedures.

RETINAL DETACHMENT

Preliminary examination of the fundus takes into account the extent of the detachment, the areas of traction and retinal breaks so that these can be accurately localised at the time of surgical repair.

The aim of surgery is to seal retinal breaks and prevent continued vitreous traction.

All symptomatic breaks need treatment, and this is done by applying cryocoagulation to the choroid, causing reaction beneath the torn retina, to seal the tear by adhesion after the layers are approximated. This approximation is achieved by indentation of the sclera using an external plomb located over the damaged retina, or an encircling strap of silicon secured around the eye just behind the affected area.

Retinal detachment may arise spontaneously in an eye which previously had normal function, but some conditions predispose to it, e.g. myopia, traction in proliferative diabetic retinopathy, and trauma. The exact nature of the detachment has to be taken into account when deciding on the method to be used in replacing it.

A retinal detachment induced by trauma usually has a break with a bullous configuration, or transgel traction from a point of incarceration of the vitreous gel with a break on either side, or less often at the opposite diameter. Cryopexy has to be placed at either side of a scleral perforation.

When vitreous haemorrhage is followed by fibrous proliferation and when transgel traction threatens retinal detachment, a vitrectomy is required to remove traction membranes, establish the site of any breaks and clear the visual axis. This is followed by an encirclement with an anteriorly placed silicon band and circumferential cryopexy. The timing of this procedure is subject to controversy: if there is a progressing retinal detachment it may be imperative to operate immediately, but a delay of 1 to 3 weeks allows the posterior vitreous to detach from the retinal surface so that its removal is safer. Any further delay permits cellular proliferation, which can rapidly aggravate the condition and make it even more difficult to treat.

ACUTE GLAUCOMA

A patient with an intraocular pressure which approaches the systolic pressure of the vessels supplying the retina is threatened with rapid and irretrievable blindness in that eye.

Such acute glaucoma must be given vigorous treatment to bring the pressure down to normal. Topical timolol 0.5% is instilled and acetazolamide 500 mg given intravenously. This is followed with topical pilocarpine 2.0% at 5-minute intervals for four instillations. If a sharp drop of pressure has not occurred within an hour, an osmotic agent is administered, e.g. oral glycerol (1 ml/kg), or intravenous 20% mannitol (7 ml/kg). If this treatment is not effective, emergency surgery is advisable.

Usually there is a good response to these measures, and planned surgery can be performed when the eye has become quiet after the acute attack. There is a strong indication for surgery, because it is the only way to overcome and prevent the recurrence of the pupil block and angle closure which precipitated the rise of pressure. If the angle, although narrow, appears unobstructed and the pressure remains controlled without the continued use of oral acetazolamide, then a further attack should be prevented by performing a peripheral iridotomy using a direct surgical approach, or with the YAG laser. The hole made in the iris permits a free flow of aqueous from the posterior chamber, where it is formed, to the angle of the anterior chamber, where it drains.

When the angle remains closed, or the pressure rises after the withdrawal of acetazolamide, a simple iridotomy will not be effective and some form of drainage operation must be chosen (probably a trabeculectomy with a tightly sutured scleral flap).

In most cases the second eye is predisposed to closed-angle glaucoma, and a prophylactic peripheral iridotomy is indicated during the same in-patient stay.

The patient will need long-term follow-up, but surgery is usually very effective and only a minority of patients require supplementary medication to keep the intraocular pressure within normal range.

Occasionally the acute attack of glaucoma has followed a few weeks after a thrombosis of the central retinal vein. In these cases open surgery should be avoided because of the risk of severe intraocular bleeding at the time of surgery or soon afterwards.

CHRONIC GLAUCOMA

This is less likely to present at an A&E department, but it is an important condition, more common than the acute form. Patients will be assessed on the basis of their visual fields, the level of intraocular pressure and the appearance of the angle of the anterior chamber as seen on gonioscopy.

Medical therapy is often effective in controlling the intraocular pressure and thus preventing or significantly delaying the continued loss of visual field. Topical pilocarpine is effective and has a long record of therapeutic safety for glaucoma, but has the disadvantage of constricting the pupil. Timolol, Propine and adrenaline can also reduce the intraocular pressure effectively without this disadvantage. Oral acetazolamide reduces the inflow of aqueous, but it has unpleasant side-effects: drowsiness and numbness and tingling in the face and extremities are frequent. Some patients are able to tolerate a combination of such therapy and to comply with it over a long period. Most patients need to be given repeated explanations until the importance of regular treatment is fully appreciated.

If medical therapy is well tolerated and effective, surgery can be set aside. In non-compliant patients, those suffering unacceptable side-effects and those in whom medical therapy is not sufficient to control the intraocular pressure to within the acceptable range, it is necessary to resort to surgery.

Chronic glaucoma is associated with inadequate drainage of aqueous from the eye, with obstruction in the trabecular meshwork of the anterior chamber angle. Surgery is designed to open up the meshwork, or to bypass it by establishing an alternative filtration outlet. Surgical laser application to the trabecular meshwork can be effective without a surgical incision. It causes a contraction at the site of application, which opens up the adjacent meshwork and increases the flow of aqueous out of the eye.

Many operations have been devised to form a permanent fistula bypassing the trabecular meshwork and establishing diffuse subconjunctival drainage. Trabeculectomy is the operation most favoured at present. As its name implies, a portion of the trabeculum is removed under a partial-thickness scleral flap. A small peripheral iridectomy is made to permit easy access of aqueous from the posterior as well as the anterior chamber to the drainage site.

By these medical and surgical measures, sometimes in combination, most chronic glaucoma can be kept under reasonable control. Patients will need to attend at regular intervals for follow-up to ensure that pressure control is maintained and that the visual field does not deteriorate. Field testing is subjective and requires skill and experience for accuracy and reliability. Automated field charting can assist in this important but time-consuming task.

PROLIFERATIVE DIABETIC RETINOPATHY

This is associated with haemorrhage from new vessels. It is always an urgent problem and becomes an emergency if visible new vessels are seen to be beginning to bleed. Immediate laser treatment can prevent further bleeding, but cannot be applied if blood obstructs the view. In the later stages laser may be used in the course of closed intraocular surgery. This includes vitrectomy to remove blood, fibrovascular tissue and membranes, to prevent further traction on the retina and to establish optical transparency so that viable retina can function usefully. The assessment and subsequent management is time-consuming and makes heavy demands on the ophthalmic units, but has been effective in reducing the disability of diabetic patients from eye disease.

VITREOUS HAEMORRHAGE

This may present to the A&E department with sudden visual loss. When it is dense, it can be difficult to establish the source of bleeding. The possibility of retinal detachment must be considered; preceding symptoms of light flashes suggest a retinal tear and may indicate its site. When the media are opaque, ultrasonography may show a detachment. Other possible aetiological factors are diabetes and hypertension, so the urine and blood pressure need checking. Traumatic vitreous haemorrhage has already been discussed.

Many vitreous haemorrhages will absorb spontaneously with recovery of good function. Detailed fundus examination is performed as soon as ophthalmoscopy is possible. Binocular indirect ophthalmoscopy is better than the direct method for fundus examination through hazy media.

Because spontaneous absorption is the rule, vitrectomy is not performed at an early stage unless there is evidence of retinal traction or detachment. Several months should be allowed to pass before the chance of natural resolution is ruled out. An exception may be made if the patient is severely disabled by haemorrhage in the only good eye.

DISCIFORM MACULAR DEGENERATION

This presents with sudden disturbance of central vision. It is preceded by sub-retinal neovascularisation near the macula with oedema or haemorrhage. Some patients are amenable to treatment with the argon laser. They are difficult to assess and need appraisal by an ophthalmologist with access to fluorescein fundus photography. This will show the area of neovascularisation, and this must be fully treated if therapy is to be effective. If haemorrhage partly obscures the area, time must be allowed for absorption, because the laser cannot be applied through blood. If the neovascularisation passes beneath the fovea, the condition is not suitable for laser treatment.

In practice, relatively few cases of macular degeneration are suitable for treatment, but in selected patients there is no doubt that function can be preserved.

CENTRAL RETINAL ARTERIAL OBSTRUCTION

This is followed by sudden and profound loss of vision in the affected eye. It is a medical emergency and the cause must be investigated. Unfortunately, very few cases recover vision. If it is due to embolism, the risk of further emboli is high and this may require urgent medical or surgical treatment. Hypertension may be a factor. The ESR is estimated with the possibility of giant cell arteritis in mind. More usually this condition affects the vessels of the optic nerve rather then the central retinal artery, but, if it is present, urgent steroid therapy is needed to prevent the second eye being affected; often there is no recovery of vision in the first eye.

CENTRAL RETINAL VEIN OBSTRUCTION

This may be manifested in hypertension, hyperlipidaemia, hyperviscosity and diabetes. These possibilities need investigation. Chronic glaucoma may be associated and this must also be investigated. If there are obvious signs of retinal ischaemia, with florid haemorrhages and exudates, prophylactic retinal laser therapy is indicated to prevent the development of iris new vessels (rubeosis), which may lead on to intractable secondary glaucoma.

Branch retinal vein occlusion is not followed by iris rubeosis and glaucoma, but laser treatment to severe retinal neovascularisation may prevent haemorrhage. Care must be taken by studying fluorescein fundus photographs to identify any newly formed anastomotic vessels and avoid applying the laser beam to them.

7

Referral and prevention

In this final chapter two matters will be considered: first the referral of patients from the A&E department and, second, action which may be needed towards prevention of injury.

REFERRAL

HOW, WHEN AND WHERE?

Once the decision to refer the patient from the A&E department has been made, there is the question of how, when and where. Many eye patients will be ambulant, others will require transport, but almost all should be accompanied, because of disability or anxiety caused by their condition.

The degree of urgency has been outlined in previous chapters, and the clinician will have to use his/her judgement in making arrangements. In the most severe cases, specialists from other disciplines should be requested to come to see the patient so that transfer can be planned in the most effective way. At the other extreme, it may only be necessary to make a written request for a routine consultation. The majority of cases need a telephoned arrangement, after which the patient is transferred with a written summary of the history, findings and treatment already given.

For most patients presenting with ophthalmic symptoms and signs the transfer will be to the ophthalmology service, and the further measures which may follow have been outlined in the preceding chapter.

Sometimes the primary referral will be to other medical or surgical disciplines. For example, patients with central retinal arterial obstruction may be referred to a general physician, cardiologist or vascular surgeon. Vascular surgery is increasingly effective in the management of ischaemic conditions. When sight is threatened, urgent referral is needed.

Optic disc oedema with visual loss, unequal pupil reactions, diplopia, or field defects are neuro-ophthalmological and may be referred to a neurologist or ophthalmologist, but some larger centres now provide a specific neuro-ophthalmological service.

Conditions around the orbit may be in the province of other surgical disciplines as well as ophthalmic, viz: maxillofacial, otorhinological, plastic, or neurosurgical. Increasingly, surgeons from these specialities will work together on the more difficult and severe conditions, with great benefit to the patient.

Remember that eye injury may be concealed by facial and lid swelling. When referring patients in whom it has not been possible to examine the eyes, report this fact so that care will be taken to do so as soon as possible, probably when the patient is under general anaesthesia.

When infants and children are injured, the possibility that this is non-accidental must be considered. Paediatricians can contribute much to the care of children attending A&E departments and should be involved early in their management.

An ophthalmologist is able to provide a rapid assessment if approached by an A&E clinician who is in doubt about correct referral of patients with visual problems. Prompt management can usually be arranged even if an onward referral is appropriate later.

SPECIAL OPHTHALMIC EXAMINATIONS

Although patients may be transferred to the care of non-ophthalmic disciplines, the ophthalmologist can still provide support in their management by special investigations repeated at suitable intervals.

Visual evoked potentials and other electrodiagnostic recordings
These may help to confirm damage to the optic nerve or visual pathways. Serial tests can show changes over a period of time, which can be most helpful in establishing a prognosis.

Orthoptic assessment
Measurements of ocular movements and binocular field may be very helpful in monitoring progress after lesions of the ocular muscles and the IIIrd, IVth or VIth cranial nerves. Surgery for residual deviations can be very effective in improving comfort and function, but is usually deferred until orthoptic reports show that the condition is static. In the intervening time a temporary prismatic spectacle correction can give relief of symptoms.

Quantitative visual field charting
This can also be important in the diagnosis and for monitoring the progress of the condition. There are many different methods available to suit particular circumstances.

PREVENTION OF INJURY

EYE INJURY IN THE GENERAL CONTEXT

There is much general publicity directed to the prevention of accidents, but surprisingly often eye injury is not mentioned. There is a tendency to consider obvious structural damage in assessing severity of injuries generally and to forget that the eye is a very important sensory organ exposed to injury. There is need to draw attention to the frequency of eye injuries, because awareness goes some way towards prevention.

Prevention must commence after recognition of the hazard. Although A&E services are involved in management after the event, blindness from trauma can best be prevented by the removal of the hazard (primary prevention). When this is not possible, attention should be drawn to the danger and how to protect against it (secondary prevention).

GENERAL MEASURES FOR THE PREVENTION OF ACCIDENTS

Action to prevent disability follows the same pattern for all kinds of injury:

Primary prevention = prevent the accident
Secondary prevention = reduce the extent of the injury
Tertiary care = minimise the long-term handicap

Prevention is based on:
1. Altering the environment
2. Education
3. Enforcement
of which the first is the most effective.

The possibility of danger should always be borne in mind and, if it is recognised, prevention can be effective if an individual or an organisation has the duty and authority to act. Experience shows that the most speedy and effective control occurs in response to military necessity or economic pressure. In other contexts too much emphasis is placed on rehabilitation after disability from injury and too little on prevention.

Domestic accidents are neglected. In the UK, the Health and Safety at Work Act 1974 has been quite effective in making clear where responsibilities lie in promoting safety, but it does not extend to the home.

The incidence of injury from a specific cause can change very quickly. This is largely due to the efficiency of preventive measures introduced as soon as a repetitive pattern is recognised. In some respects this reflects the efficiency of medical and ancilliary services in recognising the prevalence, determining the cause, alerting those responsible and establishing the means of prevention.

Those concerned with safety have to be alert to dangers and quick to recognise increased frequency. Sometimes, dangers become well known to those of us treating the injured, before there is any public awareness. We see the results of accidents and we have a concentration of experience. We must ensure that steps are taken to draw attention to the risks by notifying people in authority and by encouraging educational programmes. Warnings on television, radio, posters and labels are effective, and it may be necessary to use these media to prevent further injury and remove the hazard.

Doctors caring for the injured have a great responsibility to draw attention to dangers, and must persist in drawing attention to them until they have stimulated those legislators, manufacturers, education authorities and voluntary bodies who are in a better position to act in prevention.

Resources are limited, and, if legislative bodies are to be convinced, the justification for extra safety precautions needs to be based on considerations of costs and benefits. Sensible limits must be put on what levels of risk are acceptable. There are surprisingly wide variations in this. We are ready to accept much higher risks during sporting activities than we will accept on public transport or at work, because risks in sport are voluntary and individuals make their own decision. An annual death risk of 1:500 is often accepted. Involuntary risks are imposed by society; then a risk of 1:1 000 000 becomes unacceptable and emotions run high. These are unreasonable differences, but within this wide range there is an undoubted place for us to initiate and encourage action to prevent injury.

INDEX